D1066677

The Illustrated Guide

to

Extended Massive Orgasm

PRAISE FOR THE AUTHORS' PREVIOUS BEST-SELLING BOOK,
EXTENDED MASSIVE ORGASM

"They are breaking new ground—and, who knows, maybe Guinness world records, too—in orgasmic studies." — *San Francisco Chronicle*

"It covers everything imaginable to do with 'clitorology,' as they call it. It's easy to understand and written without frills, in correct and graphic language, with chapters on everything to do with the whole sex package, including male orgasm." — *The Sunday Times Magazine*

"Check chapter 5 for the most detailed directions to the G-spot we've ever seen." — *GQ*

"The book's detailed instructions cover how to lubricate your honey's sweet spot, how to 'anchor' the clitoris to keep it from slipping away from you, how to properly 'stroke' the clitoris with your fingers, using different speeds and motions, and what to do with your nonstroking hand." — *Playboy.com*

"What man doesn't want to please the gals? Who doesn't want more pleasure? Bodansky's book can help here and has the added joy of being funny at times...." — *The Espresso*

DEDICATION

We would like to dedicate this book to three people.

To Carl and Alice Bodansky for showing how two people can remain in love with each other for a lifetime.

To Baka Angelina who gave Vera the strength to live and love totally and to always strive for excellence.

CONTACT INFORMATION

If you'd like more information on EMO and our courses, please visit our website at *www.extendedmassiveorgasm.com* or e-mail us at *verasteve@aol.com*.

For more information on the featured artists, please visit Kim E. Black's website at *www.kimeblack.com* and Teri Sugg's website at *www.suggarts.com*.

ORDERING

Trade bookstores in the U.S. and Canada please contact:

Publishers Group West
1700 Fourth Street
Berkeley, CA 94710
Phone: (800) 788-3123   Fax: (510) 528-3444

Hunter House books are available at bulk discounts for textbook course adoptions; to qualifying community, health-care, and government organizations; and for special promotions and fund-raising. For details, please contact:

Special Sales Department
Hunter House Inc.
P.O. Box 2914
Alameda, CA 94501-0914
Phone: (510) 865-5282   Fax: (510) 865-4295
E-mail: ordering@hunterhouse.com

Individuals can order our books from most bookstores, by calling **(800) 266-5592**, or from our website at **www.hunterhouse.com**

The Illustrated Guide to Extended Massive Orgasm

STEVE BODANSKY, PH.D.,
and VERA BODANSKY, PH.D.

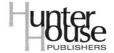

Hunter House
PUBLISHERS

Copyright © 2002 by Steve and Vera Bodansky

All rights reserved. No part of this publication may be reproduced or transmitted in any form or by any means, electronic or mechanical, including photocopying and recording, or introduced into any information storage and retrieval system without the written permission of the copyright owner and the publisher of this book. Brief quotations may be used in reviews prepared for inclusion in a magazine or newspaper or for broadcast. For further information, please contact:

Hunter House Inc., Publishers
P.O. Box 2914
Alameda, CA 94501-0914

LIBRARY OF CONGRESS CATALOGING-IN-PUBLICATION DATA

Bodansky, Steve.
The illustrated guide to extended massive orgasm / Steve and Vera Bodansky.
        p. cm.
Includes index.
ISBN 0-89793-362-1 (pb)
1. Sexual excitement. 2. Orgasm. 3. Sex instruction. I. Bodansky, Vera. II. Title.

HQ31 .B5933 2002
613.9'6—dc21   2001051975

PROJECT CREDITS

ILLUSTRATOR: Kim E. Black   ILLUSTRATOR: Teri Sugg
COVER AND BOOK DESIGN: Brian Dittmar Graphic Design
DEVELOPMENTAL EDITOR: Kelley Blewster   COPY EDITOR: Laura Harger
PROOFREADER: Rachel E. Bernstein   INDEXER: Kathy Talley-Jones
ACQUISITIONS EDITOR: Jeanne Brondino   ASSOCIATE EDITOR: Alexandra Mummery
PUBLICITY AND MARKETING: Sara Long, Earlita K. Chenault
CUSTOMER SERVICE MANAGER: Christina Sverdrup   ORDER FULFILLMENT: Lakdhon Lama
ADMINISTRATOR: Theresa Nelson   COMPUTER SUPPORT: Peter Eichelberger
PUBLISHER: Kiran S. Rana

Printed and bound by Bang Printing, Brainerd, Minnesota
Manufactured in the United States of America

9 8 7 6 5   First Edition   04   05   06

~ Contents ~

⤙ Illustrations ⤚

⟶ Important Note ⟵

The material in this book is intended to provide a review of extended massive orgasm. Every effort has been made to provide accurate and dependable information, and the contents of this book have been compiled through professional research and in consultation with medical professionals. We believe that the sensuality advice given in this book poses no risk to any healthy person. However, if you have any genital infections, such as herpes, we recommend that you consult your doctor before using this book.

The author, editors, publishers, and the professionals quoted in this book cannot be held responsible for any error, omission, professional disagreement, outdated material, or adverse outcomes that result from applying any of the information in this book. If you have questions concerning the application of the information contained in this book, consult a qualified professional.

⟶ Definitions ⟶

For a working understanding of several terms we commonly use, we recommend that you read these definitions before reading the rest of the book.

AT CAUSE: We use this phrase to refer to a state in which one only gives attention, and does not receive attention.

AT EFFECT: We use this phrase to refer to a state in which one only receives attention, and does not give attention.

COMING, ORGASM, GETTING OFF: These terms all mean the same thing: the pleasure one feels emanating from one's genitals. An orgasm can start before the first touch (or stroke) and last until after the last stroke. An orgasm triggers all or some of the following reactions, which you can observe in your partner: muscular contractions, increased heart rate, increased breathing, flushing of neck and face, engorgement of genitals, and secretion from genital glands.

DETUMESCENCE: We use this term to describe a decrease in sexual energy. In an orgasm, the term refers to the time when physical intensity is on the way down. It is synonymous with the phrases *going down* and *coming down*.

DO, DOING: This is our term for the manual stimulation of another person's genitals to produce pleasure. It includes all the mental attention, preliminary teasing, and communication skills that are necessary to produce an extended massive orgasm, or EMO.

DOEE: The doee is the person who allows someone else to control his or her nervous system to produce an orgasm; the doee is the one who is "getting done."

DOER: This is the person who produces pleasure or orgasm in another person's body.

DONE: We use this term to mean the process of giving someone control of one's nervous system, as in *being done or getting done.*

EMO (EXTENDED MASSIVE ORGASM): An orgasm of great intensity that lasts for an indefinite amount of time.

INTROITUS: The entrance to the vagina.

PEAK (n.): The highest point reached in each cycle of an orgasm. As in a mountain range, there can be many peaks in an orgasm.

TO PEAK, PEAKING (v.): To notice when the highest point of the orgasmic cycle is reached and to deliberately take the orgasm down a notch or more so that the orgasm is able to continue and rise higher on the next cycle. Also refers to the act of reaching (if you're the doee) or creating (if you're the doer) the peaks.

SENSUAL (adj.): Having to do with the five senses and conceptual thought; stimulating the senses in a pleasurable way.

SENSUALITY (n.): We use this term to indicate the effect of stimulating the body with the intention to produce pleasure. When one is pursuing sensuality, one does only what feels good at the moment.

SEXUALITY: In contrast to *sensuality,* we use *sexuality* to mean reproductive behavior: literally, sexual intercourse, when the man's penis enters the woman's vagina. The goal of sexuality is reproduction, male orgasm accompanied by the release of sperm and the meeting of the sperm with the egg.

SEXER: A person who is having sex and who has the ability to take and create pleasure in a sensual experience.

SPOT: The place on the clitoris or penis that is most sensitive in most people.

SURRENDER: The act of allowing someone else to control one's nervous system in order to experience an EMO. One is surrendering not to a superior force, as that would constitute defeat, but to one's own greater pleasure.

TUMESCENCE: Derived from the Latin word *tumor,* which means "to swell" or "to engorge." We use the term to describe an increase in sexual energy or body energy. In an EMO, the word means the intensification of energy that drives the orgasm. Synonymous with the phrase *going up.*

TURN-ON: Turn-on is when a woman is in agreement with her own desires and can stimulate a response in another person's body, either sexually or otherwise, to gratify these desires.

A Note about Language

In this book, we've usually used formal terms to refer to the sex organs and sexual acts, such as *vagina, penis,* and *ejaculate.* Occasionally, however, when it seemed to work best, we've used their four-letter equivalents. Since words such as *pussy, cock,* and *come* are the words many people use in daily life, we felt we should sometimes do the same in our books, and we mix them with more technical terms, such as *penis, vulva,* and the like. We do not wish to offend anyone, and we hope that our readers will be able to move beyond any initial disagreement or discomfort they may feel with our choice of words.

~ Acknowledgments ~

This book is the result of our years of training and teaching. We are extremely grateful to Dr. Vic Baranco and our coteachers at More for both our initial exposure to and detailed study of pleasure. For the past ten years we have been teaching and researching orgasm independently. We are grateful to all of our students who allowed us to gain even more understanding of the art of extended orgasm.

We would like to acknowledge Dr. Earle M. Marsh, M.D., for his early influence and lifelong friendship.

We are especially appreciative of the playful appetite of Regena Thomashauer, who stimulated us to create new strokes and ideas, and thank her along with her husband Bruce for their continued friendship.

We are grateful to Wendy, Francoise, Judy, and Regena for demonstrating the fun a woman can have with a penis.

We would like to thank Sherry Mueller and Kim Kyllo for their desire and appetite.

We are thankful to Shawn Mueller, Michael O'Callaghan, Karen McCarthy, Barbara Boje, and Alan Pryor for their help with the photography for the illustrations.

We are indebted to Teri Sugg (see her work at *www.suggarts.com*) for her help with the photography and for her wonderful drawings.

We are thrilled that Kim E. Black (see his work at *www.kimeblack.com*) was able to give us so much of his time and effort in creating many of the beautiful illustrations.

We would like to thank Dr. Neville Marks and Dr. Renato Sabbatini for their suggestions.

We are appreciative of the many questions that Branko, Brane, Kastelic, and Santi contributed.

We are overwhelmed by the editing that Kelley Blewster and Laura Harger were able to do to take our manuscript and make it into something readable and enjoyable. We thank the staff at Hunter House, especially Alex, Kiran, and Jeanne, who have made this project fun and seemingly effortless.

We are also grateful to the many people who have e-mailed us with their acknowledgment of how our first book added to their lives. Thank you.

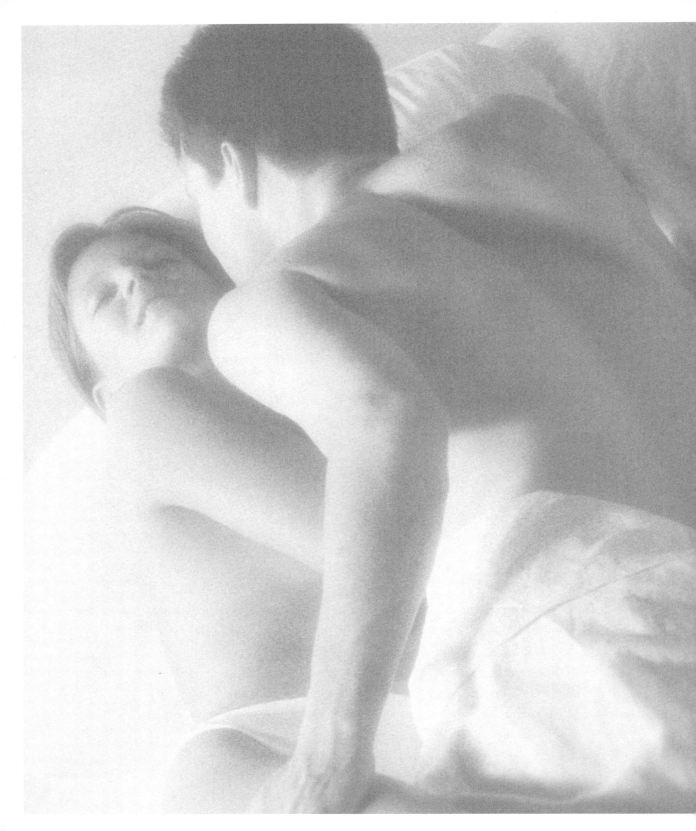

— Introduction —

Marshmallow kisses with pillows delicious.
Soft silky lips playing sweet refrain.
Tongues meet at the opening feast.
Uniting beauty with the former beast.

Pressed against your magic pillow,
Falling into your siren spell.
Captured by your wild call,
Into your heart is where I've fallen.

You are love and I'm loving you,
As long as time does flow.
If time should end, our love will not.
And we will make a new world grow.

The two of us — Steve and Vera — have been students and teachers of sensuality for a total of more than fifty years. We make sensuality and pleasure the highest priority in our lives, more important than success or anything else. This does not mean we stay in bed all the time, stimulating each other. It *does* mean that when we reach a fork in the road or have to make a decision, we choose the path that feels the most pleasurable and fun. We have both chosen "orgasm" as our field of specialization — specifically, orgasm in women — although we also study and teach about men's orgasms to both classes and private clients. We cannot think of a more pleasurable subject.

1

We believe that humans have the power to create our lives as we want them to be. We are the directors and creators of our experience. However, because of societal prejudices, it is often difficult to express the desire for pleasure, especially sensual pleasure. Our society is based on the idea that you have to pay for pleasure with the currencies of pain and work. Many religions teach that we must experience suffering here on earth if we are to experience the pleasure of going to heaven.

Yet there remains within all of us an innate desire to experience intense physical and emotional pleasure. This desire is kept from fully revealing itself by society's rules and laws. These rules, and the people defending them, have been quite successful at keeping us from realizing our true pleasure potentials. However, they have been unable to keep all the information about pleasure from leaking out. The information gathered in this book is propleasure. It is real, and it works.

Our work has been made possible by the earlier work of heroes who were able to step out of the box and notice that the emperor was wearing no clothes—and what's more, that the emperor was having a lot of fun without his clothes. Dr. Vic Baranco, pioneering sexologist and master teacher, has been our biggest hero. He created an experimental lifestyle for himself and many other pleasure seekers. He refused to accept the word *can't*. He showed us that orgasm does not have to be limited to a few seconds and a few contractions; it can begin with or before the first touch or stroke and continue throughout the whole sexual experience; it can last many minutes or even hours at ever-increasing intensities that far surpass the usual, short orgasm.

That, in a nutshell, is the definition of an *extended massive orgasm*, or EMO. Through our study and work, we have learned that EMOs are best and most efficiently produced with the hands, and we've spent many years teaching people exactly how to use their hands to produce EMOs. This book is a continuation of our teaching careers, and in it we provide many techniques, examples, and illustrations showing where and how to touch someone to produce the best orgasm.

We believe that orgasm is our birthright. After all, we were all conceived in orgasm. We also believe that EMOs are not an aberration, a departure from the "norm" of an ordinary orgasm, but can themselves be the norm. We think that eventually the words *extended* and *massive* won't have to be used when people describe an orgasm, because most orgasms will be intense and extended. The orgasm that is considered normal now will be described in the not-so-distant future by an adjective such as "short" or "sneeze-like." In our first book, *Extended Massive Orgasm: How You Can Give and Receive Intense Sexual Pleasure*, we made the analogy that if the orgasm that most people know now is like the Wright brothers' plane, then the extended massive orgasm is like the space shuttle!

We have been thrilled, if not totally surprised, at the enthusiastic response to our first book. That book—like this one—is about pleasure, and it was a pleasure to write and a pleasure to see it published. Everything involved with its production was pleasurable, even when we had to adjust our attitude to find the pleasure in the process. That just goes to show you: when you aim for pleasure, you often encounter success along the way.

Why an Illustrated Book on EMO?

Many people from all over the world have written to tell us how our first book, *Extended Massive Orgasm,* enhanced their love lives. Many of our readers have also asked for more detailed information about topics and techniques we addressed in that book. We are amazed and delighted that such a great appetite exists in the world for information about sensual pleasure and better orgasms. This book, *The Illustrated Guide to Extended Massive Orgasm,* aims to further satisfy that appetite, and through exercises, tips, new techniques, and illustrations, we hope to help our readers learn more about pleasure and how to produce it.

As we stated above, most of our research and work has focused on the sexual pleasure of women. This is, as we pointed out in *Extended Massive Orgasm,* because of the age-old prejudice that says men's orgasms are more important than women's. Before you protest that such a statement is an exaggeration, think about it. How have people traditionally defined the end of the sex act? With the man's ejaculation. Only in the last quarter of the twentieth century, with the feminist movement and the sexual revolution, did women's orgasms become an issue of importance. We feel called to contribute to rectifying that imbalance. This book builds on our last one by focusing even more thorough attention on techniques for clitoral stimulation, the source of all orgasms for women.

But we also recognize that men's orgasms need to be radically redefined. Men can expand their experience of orgasm to something far more pleasurable than a "squirt, squirt" at the end of coitus. For this reason—and because many readers of our first book want to learn techniques specifically devoted to pleasuring the penis—*The Illustrated Guide to Extended Massive Orgasm* provides a much more detailed look at male orgasm. It includes lots of information on male anatomy, on teasing a man, on teaching a man to receive an EMO, and on giving a man an EMO. There is quite a lot in the bookstores about penile stimulation. But there is not much about giving men intense, long orgasms—as we teach you how to do here. We also provide information that helps both partners enjoy the experience of stimulating the man—playing with a man's genitals is a lot of fun, for *both* partners. We have also added an entire chapter of useful ways to pleasurably detumesce both partners after an EMO.

We have included numerous techniques that we use in our private sessions with our clients. Although most of these techniques can be used by anyone interested in pleasure, a few are designed for very serious students who may wish to teach this information to others.

Our first book has created quite a stir. We hope to continue that stir with our second book, so this time we've used pictures as well as words to explain the techniques we present. But looking at the pictures and reading the words is not enough. To master the techniques, you must practice them and make them a part of yourself, just as you must practice when learning to drive a car or play a musical instrument. Once the techniques are second nature, you can take your attention off them and focus all your attention on creating fun and pleasure, using the techniques in the ways that suit you best. After all, we're not hoping to make clones of ourselves or teach everyone to pleasure each other exactly as we do. We hope people learn and practice the techniques we offer and then create their own styles, ones that work best for them.

Pleasure and sex have a bad name in our culture; even though most people continue to have sex (after all, the population continues to grow), we're all taught many reasons to fear it, from sexually transmitted diseases to unwanted pregnancies. Part of the problem is that most people define *sex* as *intercourse*. But in fact, there are many other ways to have sex, which avoid the risks associated with intercourse. Extended massive orgasm through manual stimulation of the genitals is a practically risk-free activity that can add much pleasure to one's life. And EMO also improves all aspects of sensuality; even intercourse is enhanced after one learns more about one's own body and one's partner's body.

Many people are scared of sex. Fear comes from either lack of familiarity or negative past experience. But bravery and courage come from engaging in action despite our fears. Once sensuality is practiced and embraced, fear disappears like morning mist evaporating in the sun. Sensuality—as opposed to sexuality—is about enjoying each touch and each moment. When you can keep your attention on the present during a sensual experience, you no longer worry about or fear anything else; fears about the future and anxieties from the past vanish. All your energy is on the experience, not wasted in fear or regret. Learning and practicing EMO as taught in this book enhances your ability to live fully and experience each moment as it happens.

〰 The Structure of the Book 〰

Although I (meaning Steve) typed this book, it is, like our last one, a joint endeavor. Together Vera and I have discussed all the topics that are included here, and we've gone over each sentence to make sure we agree on what we've written.

Now, on to the nuts and bolts of the book itself. We've included a list of definitions early in the book. We suggest that you read through these before reading the rest of the book so you will have a working understanding of how we use important terms.

The first chapter of this book provides an overview of the fundamentals of an EMO: what an EMO is and how it's produced. This chapter can serve as an introduction for newcomers to the concept or a refresher course for those who have read our first book, *Extended Massive Orgasm*. We recommend that beginners also read that book, however, for a comprehensive discussion of EMOs.

The second chapter, "Teasing," describes how to tease a lover, which is an essential part of producing an EMO, but also, we hope, teases the reader. This may be the most essential chapter in the book. Only when one knows how to tease—when to approach and when to back off, when to entice and when to bring down—can one control an EMO in one's partner.

To become proficient in producing an EMO, one has to know the basic structure and functioning of the genitals and learn how to touch them, so we've dedicated Chapter 3 to an in-depth exploration of the anatomy of the genitalia in both sexes. We have found in our research that the optimal way to produce an EMO is with hand-to-genital stimulation. Obviously, on a man, the penis is the organ that is most efficiently stimulated to produce pleasure. But our work also has been dedicated to teaching women and men of the importance of the clitoris, and its direct stimulation, to a woman's pleasure. Thus, we present techniques and information on the anatomy of the male and female genitals and explain where, when, and how to stimulate them for the greatest effect. Essential concepts taught in this chapter include the technique of exposing the clitoris from under its hood and an explanation of how the male ejaculatory response works.

Chapter 4, "Positions," describes and illustrates the best way to place one's hands and fingers on the clitoris or the penis for maximum effect. It also explains and depicts several different body positions for administering an EMO.

To be stimulated to an intense and extended orgasm, a person must know what kind of strokes feel best to him or her. One of the best ways to learn this is by becoming intimately familiar with one's own body. Thus we have included a chapter on masturbation. Chapter 5 outlines extremely effective exercises that can be used throughout one's life to get the most out of masturbation and fantasy.

The sixth chapter, "Receiving an EMO," is all about surrender and communication, which are both vital to experiencing an EMO. First we describe techniques for relaxation, which is an essential element of surrender. We detail the importance of expressing acknowledgment and approval of your partner. Then we explain how to get your partner to touch you just as you like, and we explain how men can teach their partners to extend their orgasms by getting close to, but not going over, the ejaculatory edge.

The next and closely related chapter is all about giving an EMO, to both men and women. The art of doing someone and giving them an EMO includes knowing how to touch and, equally important, recognizing when to stop and when to start again, which is known as peaking. This chapter explains peaking and how to communicate during the EMO, and it explains how to control your partner's nervous system. We describe specific strokes and techniques designed to take your partner as high as possible.

Chapter 8, "Pressures," discusses different levels of pressure used in sensual touch—ranging from the gentle to the playful to the firm. It includes exercises to help readers learn more about what levels of pressure they and their partners find pleasurable. And Chapter 9 provides helpful information about vaginal and anal insertion, as well as creative use of the "second hand" (the one not used for direct genital stimulation).

Our society places negative connotations on the idea of "coming down," so in Chapter 10 we demonstrate the positive aspects of this post-EMO stage of the sensual experience. We describe different methods for bringing someone to a lower state of tumescence while still maintaining a high state of pleasure.

Finally, we've included a question-and-answer section at the back of the book. Our readers really enjoyed a similar section in our first book, and this appendix allows us to answer specific questions that we have received from students and readers and to include additional pertinent information about sensuality and EMOs.

Someone once wrote to us to comment that it must be wonderful to live without stress, as we presumably did. We laughed. Choosing pleasure as one's top priority does not turn one into a yoga master who enjoys total control all the time. We experience all the normal human emotions, and sometimes we feel stressed out or even victimized by circumstance. Experiencing some stress is a necessary part of being alive. It is also possible fuel for orgasm. Orgasm is one way that our bodies can channel the energy that they produce in response to our physical and emotional environment. Living in the twenty-first century, with all our immediate access to news and information, makes it very easy for people to focus their attention on any number of negative occurrences, from crime to war. We believe that we live where our attention is placed. It is possible and extremely beneficial to our health and sanity to express our love, demonstrate the positive aspects of human relationships, and pay attention to our own pleasure and that of our loved ones. The information that you can learn from this book—and, through practice, incorporate into your life—could be the road to a life of wonderful pleasures and great intimacy.

CHAPTER ONE

Choosing Pleasure In the introduction, we said that we've made pleasure our first priority. How did we do that when, obviously, not everything in life is fun and pleasurable? We did it by getting into agreement with the events and circumstances of our lives and learning to recognize choices when they present themselves to us. Choices present themselves at every moment of our lives, and when you choose correctly, you can guide yourself toward a better, more pleasurable existence. But uncovering—the better word is recognizing—these choices often requires an attitude adjustment. That adjustment consists of getting into agreement with what is occurring in your life, for only then can you hope to move on to a higher level.

EMO: The Basics

What do we mean by the phrase "getting into agreement with what is occurring in your life"? We mean facing the reality of your life in the present moment—accepting how it *is* before focusing on how you *wish* it could be. People often get into trouble and are unhappy when their expectations outdistance their realities. As Robert Ornstein and David Sobel, authors of *Healthy Pleasures*, state, "Happiness lies in narrowing the distance between where you see yourself and where you expect to be." Here's another way to state the same idea: When you take responsibility for your life as it is *now*, you can then guide its course toward more pleasure.

In order to experience an EMO, you must first have a high awareness of and agreement with what occurs during a sensual encounter. The more positive awareness (or attention) that you can focus on the pleasure at hand, the greater your ability to expand and intensify that pleasure. Similarly, the more in agreement you are with your experience, the greater your ability to change and redirect that experience. There are two ways of getting into agreement: change your viewpoint or get things into agreement with your viewpoint. In the context of an EMO, this means learning to recognize pleasure (in other words, overcome anxiety and tension to experience the pleasure at hand) and learning to request changes that will intensify your pleasure (in other words, get things into agreement with what you want). So both "getting into agreement" methods are essential to EMOs, and both will help you learn to focus on immediate sensation, the stroking of your partner, and the pleasures of the present moment.

These are the actual mental tricks or attitudes that are basic to having an EMO. Both help you focus on the present moment rather than direct your energy toward some future goal of even better stimulation. It's fine, and sometimes even necessary, to think ahead toward increased feelings of pleasure, but to get there, your immediate response to your present sensations must be one of approval and agreement. This might seem paradoxical, but an EMO is a sensual experience, and that means that it happens one stroke at a time, one moment at a time: the only time you should think about is the "right now." Making this change in your perception will also broaden your conception of what is possible, and with that mental expansion, your pleasurable sensations will expand accordingly.

We frequently are asked the question "Why have an EMO?" Sometimes we facetiously answer, "Because it is there. It's like climbing Mount Everest." But the true answer touches upon many reasons. One does not have to have an EMO to live, of course. It is a luxury, but it is perhaps the greatest luxury that one can have. It costs you, and the price is time, but it is time spent in pleasure. The results are not only better orgasms but better communication skills and greater intimacy with one's partner. And by learning to be in present time while experiencing an EMO, one learns to take this ability into the rest of one's life, resulting in more joy and bliss and less fear and worry. Women and men who have experienced an EMO often become nicer and more generous, and women and men who can produce an EMO often grow more confident in all aspects of their lives. And, of course, the immediate pleasure of having and giving an EMO is the highest level of physical and emotional gratification that is available in life.

The knowledge that an EMO is possible and obtainable is also vitally important to having one. It is best to approach this subject with a beginner's mind. Many people have such a fixed idea of what an orgasm is and how it looks that they totally dismiss the very idea of—and thus the possibility of experiencing—an EMO. Their dismissal is due in part to the fact that many of the physical signs of an EMO, its observable bodily responses, include signs that most people equate with symptoms of ordinary sexual arousal. But there is a difference, and it's a profound one. In an EMO, the doee is relaxed, has surrendered his or her nervous system, and is totally focused on the exquisite "orgasmic" sensation that starts with or even before the first stroke. That concept of "surrender" is difficult for many people, who equate it with being a victim, which is usually considered a negative predicament. Surrender opposes our usual view of life, in which we're always responsible for and in control of everything. But to experience the highest orgasm one actually has to completely give up control of one's nervous system to someone else, to surrender to the pleasure being produced. This is a highly vulnerable, even "victimized" state, yet it's the only way to receive the optimum orgasm. To be a pleasure victim is the best and, indeed, the only possible route to the highest pleasures.

EMOs Versus "Normal" Orgasms

The old, usual view of orgasm is pretty simple. A person tenses up his or her body, continually focusing on the squirt or release that comes at the end of sex. And thus the person misses out on most of sensuality, on all those pleasurable sensations found along the way, to reach what we like to call a "crotch sneeze," an orgasm lasting perhaps ten or so seconds. An EMO, on the other hand, is like an ocean with waves that continually roll with ever-increasing intensity. To those who have never experienced an EMO, such an orgasm might seem impossible. But as we said above, just gaining the knowledge that this type of orgasmic experience is available has opened up and freed numerous students to enter this new realm of intense and extended ecstasy.

Many people confuse male ejaculation with an orgasm, and ejaculation indeed can be *part* of an orgasm. It is the end to a sexual experience; it is the coming down and release of tumescence. But it's only the tip of the iceberg of orgasm. A man who is relaxed and enthusiastically focused on immediate pleasurable sensations may seep or ooze ejaculate for long periods of time and extend his orgasm well beyond what he believed possible. The outdated view of male orgasm also affects women: For years women have tried to imitate men's "ejaculation orgasm" by tensing their bodies to a point of no return, at which the built-up pressure had to be released all at once. A woman experiencing EMO, on the other hand, is relaxed. Tension is not part of the equation. This is why any person—male or female—who wants to have an EMO must be relaxed throughout the period of genital stimulation.

This book discusses EMO technique in even more detail than our first book does, yet it is about far more than just technique. Fun is the goal of a sensual experience, as opposed to how long or intense an orgasm you can have. However, when you do have a long and intense orgasm you usually also have fun. Some people worry that they do not have enough extra time in their days to give or receive an hour-long orgasm. In one course we teach, called DEMO (demonstration of an extended massive orgasm), we show a woman in orgasm for an hour, but we do this only to demonstrate what is possible. In the normal routine of our life, a fifteen- or twenty-minute orgasm is more usual. Even a five-minute orgasm is gratifying.

"Doer" and "Doee": The Roles in an EMO

Learning to give and receive EMOs requires training and practice, and we recommend that partners divide up their roles—one person becomes the doer, and the other, the doee. This helps attain optimum orgasmic potential. The person receiving the EMO has to surrender and become a "pleasure victim," and the person giving the EMO has to take full control and complete responsibility for the experience. These roles are not static and may change: partners can do each other in turn, or they can take turns being doer and doee in different encounters.

If you are the doee, you know that you're having an EMO when you are relaxed, when you're focusing all your attention on the immediate sensation and the pleasure you feel in your genitals, and when each successive stroke feels better and better. You are able to feel this pleasure and blissful state in your genitals for periods of time far surpassing your previous experiences. The intensity of the orgasm increases over time with practice and with approval from your partner.

If you're the doer, you realize that you are producing an EMO in your partner by the pleasure that you feel in your hands and body while doing it. You can feel that your partner is relaxed and going for every bit of sensation possible. You can feel the contractions and the orgasm increasing. You're touching the doee for your *own* pleasure—that is an essential part of giving

an EMO. You touch as if you were touching a piece of velvet or soft fur. We sometimes refer to this way of touching as the "velvet touch." The velvet touch is that stroke that feels best to the doer as well as to the doee.

Whether you are the doer or the doee, communication between both partners must be constant. If a touch feels less than great, communicate that fact; if it feels great, communicate that fact, too.

What's Love Got to Do with It?

When two people are in love with each other, they have a great foundation on which to build a life of sensual joy. And love grows best when it's fed and watered. The food and water that we are talking about are great communication and curiosity. Interest, good communication, and affection make the sensation of an EMO go higher, but they also make the relationship go higher. Love is not a static emotion; it rises and falls. To keep it going up, you have to stay in communication with and pay lots of attention to your partner.

However, to have or produce a great orgasm, you do not have to be in love with your partner. You *do* have to love what you are doing. Communication and attention are still of utmost significance. We have known students who wanted to master the techniques that we offer yet did not have steady partners with whom to practice. Some of them made an agreement to have sensual dates with another interested student; together, they practiced the information they learned from our courses. Sometimes this research lasted for only a few sessions, but other times, these relationships developed into lifelong love affairs.

We believe that love is manifested (in other words, created) by positive attention. The more positive attention that you focus on someone or something, the more love you will both feel and demonstrate. The ability to be in the present moment, up-to-date communications, and touching with confidence and enjoyment are all equally important in creating an EMO and in creating a love relationship. This is where the technique comes in. In order to be able to produce an extended massive orgasm in another body, you will have to put an extended massive amount of attention on that person. The techniques and information that we will be presenting in this book will allow you to best be able to do that. The skills for creating and receiving an EMO are fairly simple but are best when practiced until they have become second nature. Once the techniques are ingrained, you can develop your own style and flair.

Vera and I are prime examples of what can happen between two interested students of sensuality. It is our love for each other that has caused us to want to explore a path of deep intimacy in the physical, mental, and spiritual realms. Our two books and our coaching of individual students would have been impossible if our love for each other were less intimate. The techniques presented in this book are primarily in physical and mental ones. We describe ways to position your hand, how to relax your body, and what to do to produce an EMO. We discuss the importance of excellent communication. However, the spiritual plane—although not directly involved in these techniques—is actually the surrounding ethos from which these physical and mental techniques emerge. Our love for each other is what makes the rest possible.

〜 Boredom 〜

An old adage states that if you put a coin in a jar for every sex act a couple engages in during their first year of marriage, and then took a coin out for every sexual act after that, you would never empty the jar. For most couples, their sex lives become less and less fun. When people fall in love, they experience a "chemistry," or hormonal effect, that can last for a few years. This produces what we call "turn-on" and enables the couple to pursue pleasure. Turn-on is when a woman is in agreement with her own desires and can stimulate a response in another person's body—either sexually or otherwise—to gratify these desires. The female of all mammals is the sex that goes into heat. The male is able to respond to this heat but not able to initiate it directly. In her book *Love Scents*, Michelle Kodis describes this ability of women in terms of pheromones that can influence human behavior. Whether it is pheromones alone or a combination of pheromones and other senses such as visual, olfactory, and auditory that transmit the turn-on is not fully understood. Once the chemistry wears off, it becomes necessary that the couple have good communication and sound sensual techniques that they practice together in order to keep their sensual life exciting and fulfilling.

When we are kids, we can repeat the same experience or listen to the same story over and over without getting bored. Each experience is unique and new. As we get older, we become jaded. We won't watch a movie that we saw ten years ago because it is not new. We have the same partner in bed each night, but we don't want to do the same old things with them once again. We call ourselves *bored*. According to James Gleick in the book *Faster: The Acceleration of Just About Everything*, "boredom" is a recently invented word. Samuel Johnson said in the 1600s, "To be born in ignorance with a capacity of knowledge, and to be placed in the midst of a world filled with variety, perpetually pressing upon the senses and irritating curiosity, is surely a sufficient security against 'the languishment of inattention.'" Boredom is the languishment of inattention.

When we are making love, we often fail to pay continual attention. We are in our heads, wondering what the other person is thinking and comparing our sensations to previous ones. The two key words that Johnson uses are *attention* and *curiosity*. If we actively cultivate these qualities, we can enjoy every single sexual act with our steady partners. Johnson was right when he said that we have the capacity for these qualities, but he was wrong when he assumed that merely having this capacity is a sufficient security against boredom. We have to be sure to *employ* this capacity. To ensure an enjoyable experience, we must remain conscious and do only what feels good to us at each moment. People get bored because they are boring. If you do not want to be bored, then become more curious about, involved in, and fascinated by what you are doing.

Identity and Limitations

The identity of a human being is determined by the sum of all his or her limitations. Here, *limitations* is not a negative term; it means the limits, boundaries, or characteristics people embrace in all areas of life, whether physical, such as height and weight, or social, such as education, religion, or relationship status. We might describe someone as a six-foot-two-inch heterosexual male surgeon with blue eyes, who is married, has two children, plays the piano, and played basketball in college. Another person might be identified as a five-foot-four-inch female personal trainer and nutrition counselor with two children and no husband. These are just two people and only a few of their characteristics or limitations are listed. If we were to describe all their limitations, they would become completely identified, and their uniqueness or differences from anyone else would become that much more apparent. If people's limitations did not vary, then everyone would be the same. Limitations are what make us unique.

There are two ways of acquiring new limitations or adding to our identity. One is conditioning and the other is training. *Conditioning* means adding new limitations without signing up for the course, so to speak. Conditioning happens as we conform to the wishes of our parents, our peers, and other social forces. It happens as we adopt certain rules and behaviors to become a member of a given society. You may not care what kind of clothes you wear, but when everyone around you is wearing blue jeans, you probably will find yourself wearing blue jeans, too. Through conditioning, you learned to use the toilet and to wipe your backside with toilet paper. Before there was paper, children were conditioned to use leaves and twigs or their left hands, and to do it outside the cave. Such rules and behavioral expectations differ according to where and when you live. They differ from one part of a country to another, and, more obviously, from country to country.

The rules that we have adopted in our home society have enabled most of us to survive. In fact, these rules were all created for reasons of survival. Some were made simply to keep Mom and Dad from getting pissed off.

Others were made to keep you out of jail. Some were made to prevent ridicule. The rules and your behavior change continually as you grow up and grow old, even if you never leave your place of birth.

Guilt results when you follow one of your rules and then judge your behavior by another of your rules. You don't like your behavior because of that second rule, so you feel guilty for having behaved in that way. You may have yelled at your children for making irritating noises because you have a behavioral response or rule whereby certain levels of sound drive you mad; then you may later feel guilty because you have a rule against yelling at your children.

We have rules for every imaginable situation. We have so many rules for behavior that we can usually choose among the vast assortment of them and still fit into most situations. For example, we speak differently when we hang out with our teenage friends than we do when we have dinner with our grandparents. For the most part, we are not tied down to any rigid behavior; we are free to engage in different social games. The more conscious you become of your rules and your behaviors, the more you are able to take advantage of opportunities to change them and select among them.

It is very important to understand that even though our conditioning seems to have been thrust upon us, we nevertheless do have a choice in whether to agree or disagree with it. Most people (especially teenagers) do not do everything that their parents tell them to do. Even among adults, there is always someone who refuses to follow everyone else and simply won't wear those blue jeans. Realizing that we do have choice can be either very freeing or very painful. It is freeing because we realize that we are each responsible for creating our own unique set of choices and behaviors. We are each responsible for what we have done and where we are. There is very little room for blame here, so if you have blamed others for your circumstances — such as your parents or the government — it can become painful to find out that it was really your own doing all the time. Again, the choice is yours: you can view this responsibility as freeing, or you can feel that you've "lost" because of it. In this book, we do not ask you to give up any of your rules;

we *do* ask you to notice which of your rules work best for you under each set of circumstances.

Besides conditioning, the second way of adding new limitations to our identity is *training*. When we want to become better at anything, we find something or someone outside of ourselves—such as a book, a course, or a teacher—and assign that thing or person the power to help us change our identity, to help us add some new limitation. For example, if you want to learn to play the piano, you take piano lessons or follow an instructional video or book. As you learn, you become more limited in the way you approach the piano. To play well, you can't just touch any old key; you have to touch only certain keys, and touch them in a certain order.

The better we get at anything, the more limited we become. This is not to say that we can't adopt our own styles and exercise creativity, but as our skill improves, we become more disciplined—we won't adopt just any old style, but a more specific style, a variation upon what we have learned. Sometimes our students get upset when we say that they become more limited when they learn something new, but limitations in this context are the positive kind. In actuality, the limitations and discipline learned in any endeavor allow us more freedom and creativity.

Here's another example. Consider how you learn a new sport. If you take up tennis, you learn that you cannot hold the racket just anywhere if you want to become good at the game. You must hold its handle in a very specific way, and you must swing it using very specific motions. You must stand in a very specific position and bend your knees in a certain way. When you toss the ball in the air for a serve, you must toss it at a specific height, angle, and distance from your body. As you can see, the better you wish to become at tennis, or anything else, the more limited your choices are.

Since our identity is tied up with all our limitations, it can be challenging to change our identity. That is why we usually use an outside, "expert" source to gain new limitations and hence a different identity. This is also true when you're learning to receive and create extended massive orgasms. To reach a higher level of intimacy, you have to learn (in other words, to be trained) about communicating while making love. To experience intense orgasm, you have to let someone into your personal space (which is defined by your life-long conditioning) and to surrender your nervous system to that person. To become a better sexer (to have the maximum ability to take and create pleasure in a sensual experience), you have to go outside yourself to find appropriate information and instruction, whether it's from a book, a course, a video, or a lover.

We have been that outside source for many people, and we hope that you are able to use our expertise to help you reach your sexual goals. You were not born with an owner's manual on how best to give and receive sensual and sexual pleasure. We hope this book serves as your manual for obtaining great pleasure and fantastic orgasms.

CHAPTER TWO

The ability to tease—to know when to go close to your partner and when to step back, when to take your partner higher and when to bring your partner down—is the main requirement for those who are great at seduction and great at doing. Exercising the ability to tease is similar to practicing the martial arts, in which you use the force of your opponent as a weapon against them—only in sensual teasing, you use this force or energy as a way to take your partner to higher pleasurable sensations.

Teasing

Teasing, like seduction, is a dance. It involves going toward your partner and then backing off. It means noticing when the optimum sensation has been reached and when it might be time to move away. It requires being aware of the energy level between you and your partner and noticing which direction it is flowing. Teasing means playing as close to the edge as you can get.

The difference between teasing and torture is that teasing offers hope and promise of a happy outcome, while torture affords no hope or promise of light at the end of the tunnel. The goal of teasing is to get someone to come closer to you. It is to get that person to salivate, to anticipate future pleasure. To be good at teasing, you must closely focus your attention on your partner. You have to know when your partner has had enough teasing and wants your finger on his or her "spot" (the place on the clitoris or penis that is most sensitive). When you wait too long to touch or to verbally communicate your intention, you can create a feeling of torture in your partner.

When it comes to pleasure, we often say that women come first. This is because, throughout modern history, women's orgasms have been considered secondary to those of men, and we hope, through our teaching and books, to equalize this situation and to point out—to both sexes—the beneficial aspects of female orgasm. In our research, we've found that the couples who practiced "women first" in pleasure had the best relationships and were the most gratified. The reasons for this? Men are generally valued most for their productive abilities, and women are valued for their ability to attract and to have appetites for the production of men. The ability to please someone is a form of production: the man is producing an orgasm. Similarly, the ability to be pleasured is a form of appetite: the woman is enjoying the orgasm that the man produces for her. The production and enjoyment of orgasm, focusing first upon the woman, is the most beneficial way that men and women can relate to each other.

So, readers may be surprised that in this chapter we will describe how to tease a man before we get around to how to tease a woman (however, many tips apply to both sexes, so read through both sections for the maximum amount of information). We do this for two reasons. The first is that men cannot take as much teasing as women, and the second is that describing men's pleasure first is a way to tease our women readers. So, women are still coming first! We have also included a brief section on same-sex relations (this section focuses on observations and principles rather than on techniques; for same-sex teasing techniques, see the applicable section on teasing a man or teasing a woman) and a section on techniques for lubricating the genitals of both sexes.

Teasing a Man

A woman can usually take more teasing than a man—at least sexual teasing. Men are, in general, very goal-oriented, and anything that separates them from the goal is an obstacle. Therefore, when you're teasing a man's genitals, it is ever so important that you let him know what you are up to. Communicate verbally that you are in control and will get to his spot when you are good and ready to get there. The more you can inform your partner, the doee (male or female), about what you are up to, the more willing they'll be to surrender their nervous system into your hands. Your communication skills, confidence, and technical knowledge, as well as your curiosity, intention, attention, and creativity, all help your partner surrender. You want your partner to surrender to the most pleasure possible, not to some outside force by which they are defeated. They are surrendering to pleasure, not to you. Their surrender will look like desire. Their resistances will disappear, and the only kind of victim they will become is a pleasure victim.

Teasing, if done correctly, is all pleasure. A woman can make her partner feel pleasure just by thinking about him in relation to her pussy. She can make a man's penis hard simply by imagining it hard. A woman can flirt outrageously with a man, turn him on, and leave him feeling great. She does not have to do anything more than she wants to; if she wants only to flirt and turn him on, that is fine. Trouble comes if a man thinks he will get something else, but all she wants to do is flirt. This is sometimes called "prick teasing," but at times it can be more torture than tease. Men who are "undercomed" (in other words, haven't recently had sexual relations) and need attention are more likely to feel torture when they're teased than men who are less needy. A woman does not have to give up flirting, but to avoid making the man feel she is leading him on, she does well to make clear that this is as far as she wants to go. By paying close attention, she can notice what effect she has on the man she is flirting with and consider whether her actions are enjoyable to him or are making him crazy.

Besides flirting for the sake of flirting, a woman can deliberately use her flirtatiousness to titillate and arouse a man as a prelude to giving him an EMO; she can get him hard before she even touches him. Sometimes a woman has no problem flirting and turning a man on—until she gets into bed with him. Then her doubts, whether about her attractiveness or her past "failures," may creep into her mind and cause problems. A woman in this predicament is best advised to put her attention back on the fun and on the pleasure emanating from her clitoris. She can doubt those nasty doubts, and then start fresh.

A woman who is having fun and creating turn-on for her partner can make his penis move and grow in any direction she desires. She can create a dance by moving her hands around his penis without actually touching it. We call this maneuver the "Snake Charmer." She points her finger close to his penis and makes it follow her hand. Soon she has her man aching for her touch. As long as she maintains up-to-date communication, she can continue to tease. She can brush her hand near his genitals and even against his penis to let him know that she knows where she is going. She can then withdraw her hand and tease him more. If she knows which of her body parts turns her partner on, she can expose it, "flash" him with it. Some men like breasts, and some like butts, legs, or the pussy itself. A woman who admits her own turned-on thoughts and takes responsibility for turning her partner on raises the level of both her own and her partner's experience.

Effective teasing does not mean that a woman has to get her partner hard before she touches him. She can also make him hard using pleasurable touches. Once he starts feeling good, a man does not question whether he was engorged and turned on before he was touched or whether he got that way afterward.

If a woman is considering dressing up in lingerie and sexy boudoir outfits, we advise her to do it for herself. If she feels sexy and turned on when she's dressed a certain way, she passes that feeling on to her partner. However, if she dresses up just for the effect on her man and fails to enjoy herself, he probably won't even notice her effort. What can a woman choose to wear? A lot of men like a woman in high heels. They make her legs look shapelier and lift her buttocks. However, if she relies on high heels just to turn him on and does not enjoy wearing them—in other words, does not take responsibility for the turn-on—the effect of the high heels will be limited. Exposing body parts and wearing sexy clothes are options that a woman should use only to add to what she is already doing. They are not a necessary part of teasing or producing an EMO in a man.

As we noted, men can take only so much teasing before they get crazed. If you wish to lengthen the teasing time, it is important to let him know what you are up to, at least to some extent. You might tell him that you can feel him craving your touch, that you are deliberately doing this to him, and that, if he behaves himself, you eventually will touch him all over. You can stroke him lightly on the thighs, nipples, or belly. Or play with his pubic hair, using light strokes to tumesce him. You can use the back of your hand to lightly touch his scrotum and the area beneath it. You can gently tease the scrotum by either pulling slightly backward on its skin or grasping the scrotum behind the testicles and pulling outward, away from the body (do not press hard on the testicles themselves or push inward toward the body, as that hurts); then you can put your fist or palm under the scrotum and put pressure on his "hidden cock" (see Chapter 3, "Genital Anatomy," for an explanation of the hidden-cock area, and see FIGURE 2.1 for an illustration of this technique). Talk to him while you do this; let him know how good he feels in your hands. Let him know that although he is not inside your pussy, you feel pleasure there, and that the pleasure you feel is because of him.

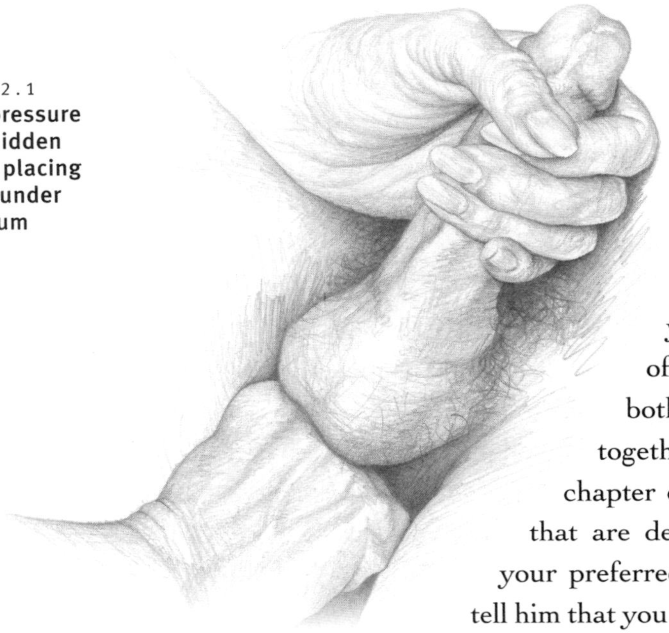

FIGURE 2.1
Putting pressure on his "hidden cock" by placing your fist under his scrotum

You can put his penis in your hand without stroking it, and then apply pressure. It's best to simply hold it at first, waiting until your own hand starts to feel good, and then to incrementally add more pressure, depending on what feels best to you. (To determine what amount of pressure in touching feels best to both of you, it's a good idea to train together beforehand. Check out the chapter entitled "Pressures" for exercises that are designed to help you learn about your preferred levels of pressure.) You might tell him that you will hold his penis for a while and probably will start stroking later, when you are ready.

Having his penis held could take his tumescence down a level. Whether that happens depends upon your intention—if you intend for him to come down and if you focus your attention on that goal, he will; if you intend for him to go up, he will. Notice which way the energy moves in your own body, and remember that you are free to do whatever feels good to you.

While doing your partner, you can stop at any point, back off a little, and tease him into wanting more and going higher when you begin touching him again. Your man is likely to love it if you take him higher with stroking and then hold his penis, and maybe squeeze it, for however long you choose. As we have stated, men tend to be focused on the goal, which to most men is ejaculation. Play with his attention; get him to feel what you are doing to him in the moment. You might even tell him that if he doesn't stop focusing on his squirting and pay attention to what you are doing right now, he will never get there. Let him know that you are the one in charge of when and whether he squirts.

Play with his fantasies. Verbally fantasize about the various sexual acts that you might do to him. If you know of certain women who are sexually appealing to him, you can introduce them or their body parts into his imagination. Have them do anything you want to him that will turn him on more. You can even tease him and say that you will kick them out now, or you can bring them back later, depending on his level of surrender. However, play with his fantasies only if you enjoy them, too. If you feel pissed off or threatened by his thinking about another woman's body, even though you are holding his penis, don't introduce that type of fantasy unless you want to learn to enjoy it.

A woman who is really turned on—who really desires a man's penis—is totally irresistible. He may have previous conditioning against doing something she wants; however, a woman's turn-on is her trump card—there is no way he can resist her, in spite of any protests he may attempt. If a man does protest, a woman must stand her ground, for any retreat into doubt or anger will squelch his desire. A man is really easy when you have your hand around his erect penis. He will do almost anything you want, so take the opportunity to make him lie still and let you have your way with him. Tease him to any point that you feel will add to his pleasure. But you must enjoy the teasing yourself; otherwise, there is no reason to do it. Teasing is a way that you can have more fun, play with your turn-on, and give a man more pleasure than he has dreamed of.

Teasing a Woman

Unlike a woman, who can turn a man on just by thinking about it, a man typically is unable to turn a woman on in the same way. However, she can and will turn herself on if she's given adequate reasons to do so. A man can flirt with a woman by putting his attention on her, noticing her, and playing with her. He can tease her by offering her goodies; if she does not enthusiastically take them, he can tease her by withdrawing the offer. The game of seduction is all about noticing whether she comes toward you or moves away. If she is going away, push her away farther and faster than she was originally going. Think through all the reasons why she could refuse your offer, whatever that offer might be (perhaps you've asked her for a "do" date and she's said no); then, when she hits you with one reason, agree with her reasons and think up even bigger and better ones. Make up more reasons that she might refuse your offer, and then counter those with reasons that in actuality she could accept your offer. This switching from "reasons for" to "reasons against" keeps her off balance and also shows that your attention is focused on her. This is the seduction technique that we call "push/pull," and, if you employ it long enough, you will overcome her resistance. (You can find more push/pull ideas in the "Commonly Asked Questions" section at the back of the book.) If, on the other hand, you sense that she is coming toward you, acknowledge her presence and make more offers; pull her even closer.

Teasing has to be fun for the person doing it as well as the person receiving it. The main reason you tease your partner is to encourage her to come toward you, mentally and physically. A woman sometimes might get naked and say she wants to have sex but remain closed off and unreceptive. With just the right amount of teasing, you can get her to open up and come toward you. This means teasing with words as well as with your hands. Once you have her in bed, you can position your finger in the air above her clitoris, without touching it, and ask her to feel it. Say things such as "I may not get to your clitoris at all today," "I think I'll just rub on your inner lips and get close but not touch your clitoris," or "Your pubic hair looks so good. I'll play with that for a few minutes and may never get to your clitoris." At first, avoid touching her anywhere — not even on her pubic hair or her lips. Simply tell her what you will do to her clitoris. Even though you are not touching her clitoris, you are putting attention on it and causing her to feel it and to want you. The more you can get her to want you, the more able she'll be to surrender to you once you do start touching her.

BEGGING FOR FUN ⤞ Sometimes it's fun to make the person who is being pleasured — the doee — beg to be touched or beg you not to stop. This is usually more effective with women doees than men, because men rarely resist, so begging would just be redundant. A man who is begging may worry about looking kind of foolish—although this may be less of a concern in special circumstances. By contrast, a woman who resists pleasure and holds out and then is coerced into begging for something she really wants can turn her average orgasm into a remarkable one.

It is not always easy to get a woman to a place where she will beg for pleasure. She has to feel your confidence and realize that you will not touch her unless she asks for it with enthusiasm. When she asks or begs for your touch, you have to feel her true desire and to notice whether she is just saying the words or is really feeling them. Let her know how close she is to hitting the mark, and when she does hit the mark, reward her surrender with abandon. You can request that she beg either when she is resisting you or when she is going up. Tell her that you don't feel much, so if she wants you to continue, she has to convince you of her true desire. You might also stop on the way up, when you know she is experiencing pleasure, and tell her that she is doing well. You want her to voice her desire so she can go even higher. She is more likely to get into agreement with begging when she knows how good she can feel. However, she may not want to beg at all, especially when she strongly resists. You have to follow through on your requests; if you are not ready to stop and she won't beg you to continue, be careful about applying this technique. It is not to be used on every woman, and definitely not every time, but begging can be a lot of fun for everyone involved if it's done with style and integrity.

THE SCENIC PATH ⋘ Women generally like to feel that you are taking your time in pleasuring them. They do not want to feel that you are rushing to their genitals or clitoris. Women are less goal-oriented than men; they prefer to take the "scenic path"—the most pleasant way from point A to point B. Men usually opt for the most efficient and fastest route. It's a good idea, when doing a woman, to start by talking with her and playing with her thoughts and feelings. When a guy goes straight for a woman's genitals, we call it "crotch diving." Every once in a while a woman is so tumesced, so ready, that crotch diving is appropriate, but that is rather unusual. A slow, scenic path to her clitoris is usually the preferred route.

Along the scenic path, you can play wherever you like, as long as you have your partner's agreement (this applies to pleasuring both women and men). Play with your partner's breasts and nipples or (facial) lips. All these places contain erectile tissue; with the right pleasurable stimulation, they can become engorged. Depending on how long you'll touch a certain spot, you might want to use lubricant (see details on choosing and applying lubricants later in this chapter). Or ask your partner to wet her lips herself with her tongue. Then you can move one or all of your fingers around her lips, choosing a "focal point" on her mouth and touching her lips everywhere except the focal point, until she greatly desires your touch on that spot. You can use fast strokes or slow, lingering ones.

The lips are only one stop on the scenic path; you can have fun from the tips of her toes to the top of her head. Once you have reached the clitoris and genital area, however, keep in mind that you probably do not want to wander much to other, more distant body parts.

As you move along the scenic path, keep in mind that, when touching any of your partner's body parts, it's important to touch for your own pleasure. Your touch feels best to your partner when it's done with your own pleasure in mind, and, of course, it benefits you, the doer, to touch in such a manner. Chapter 1 of this book explains this concept in more detail, but it's a lesson worth repeating here.

Perhaps by being around women and learning about the pleasures of the scenic path, men, too, can learn to be more pleasure-oriented. Men have a goal-oriented approach to life that's useful in many circumstances, and we are not saying that men should give it up. However, when it comes to sensual experience, pleasure is a higher priority than success or goal attainment.

FEELING THE FIRST STROKE: THE SHORT SESSION

Sometimes your goal might be that your partner feel intense sensations right from the start. One of the benefits of EMO training is that it enables you to get off with the first stroke. Usually, when you get a naked man into bed and you have your hand on his joystick, he is unable to resist you, especially if you are turned on. On the other hand, a woman naked in bed—even if you have your hand on her genitals—still might hold out. If this happens often, you can do very short sessions with her. We have done sessions with students in which we give them just one or two strokes. We let them know this in advance. We still take time to tease and to play with their tumescence; then, when it is time for the first stroke, we tell them to feel as much as they can. A one-stroke session is usually very memorable; a person often has a lot to report about just one stroke.

There are other ways to conduct a short session. You can decide before-hand that the whole session will last for just five minutes. Tease your partner by asking how much of those five minutes she wants devoted to attention to her clitoris. She may choose "crotch diving" under these circumstances, but don't let her forget who is in charge. This kind of training is very beneficial to women who want to learn how to get off on the first stroke and who want their resistances to be overcome.

When I do a woman for the first time, I often notice that very little heat is coming from her genital area. This indicates that a lot of energy is getting stuck at her neck or somewhere in her abdomen. (Usually, this isn't a prob-lem with male doees: men often are more accustomed to having orgasms, so there's less fear and apprehension involved.) If you notice this happening, position your hand a few inches above her head and neck area and then tell her to bring her energy down to her pussy; at the same time, slowly move your hand in that direction. This causes her energy to flow downward. Let her know that she does not have to work at anything; the energy will flow naturally. During your manual journey from head to crotch, if you notice any areas of coolness—a blockage of heat flow—stop there, and tell her to send that energy down to her pussy or clitoris. When she releases the energy, tell her that she is doing great, that you can feel the energy and heat moving downward. Once you get to the magic land, hold your hand just above her genitalia and intend that she feel it. You can ask her to give you even more energy. The more often you do someone, the more willing she will be, if you are good at it, to send that energy downward, and you won't have to request that she do it.

TEASING TOUCHES ✧ Before you even touch your partner, you can have her "feel" your hand. Simply point at her clitoris with your finger and ask her to feel it. Or blow air at her genitals. Stroke the air just over her clitoris and the rest of her vulva. Report anything that you notice happening to her body or to yours as you do this.

Next, add your teasing touches. Put your hand on her pubic area, and let her know how good it feels and that her clitoris has to wait. Use light, circular strokes on her pubic area; feel her hair tickle your entire hand, up to your wrist and forearm (FIGURE 2.2). You can stroke her pubic hair with any side of your hand and forearm at any speed you pre-

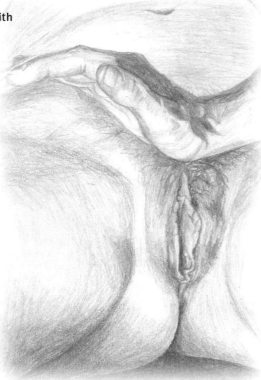

FIGURE 2.2
Teasing her pubic hair with your wrist

fer; you can move up and down or whichever way feels best. You can stroke all of your fingertips across her or use one fingertip at a time to sensually touch her pubic hair (FIGURE 2.3). Do whatever feels best to your hand. Always let her know what you are doing and how much fun it is. If you notice any wetness, engorgement, or contractions in her genitals, be sure to report them to her.

It is fun, too, to tease her inner labia. After putting some lubricant there (see below for a discussion of lubricants), move one or two fingers up and down her labia. Notice how smooth and wonderful they feel, and

report this to her. You can do one side
at a time or both labia simultaneously.
Check out different speeds and pressures. Notice any sensation in your
fingers; also notice those areas on
her lips, top or bottom, where she
feels the most sensation. You can
tease her by getting close to the
bottom of her clitoris and then
sliding your finger back downward. Let her think that the next
time you will touch her clitoris,
and then back off again at the last
second. Do this as long as it is fun.
You can go between the lips, too,
and play with her introitus in the
same manner.

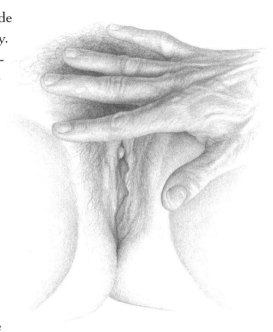

FIGURE 2.3
**Teasing a
woman's
genitals by
pleasurably
playing with
her pubic hair**

I like to approach the clitoris from the introitus and labia, slowly
working my finger upward. When I have almost reached the bottom of the
clitoris, I either linger there or retreat. It is best to talk while you are doing

this; let her know that
you know where you
are going, but that you
are not quite ready to
go there yet. Play, have
fun, and tease her by
saying, "This is as
good as it may get."
You can try a stroke
we've nicknamed the
"Michael Douglas" stroke,
after some of his movie

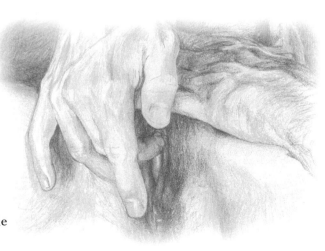

FIGURE 2.4
**The "Michael
Douglas"
stroke**

FIGURE 2.5
Using your finger to tease the clitoris through the hood

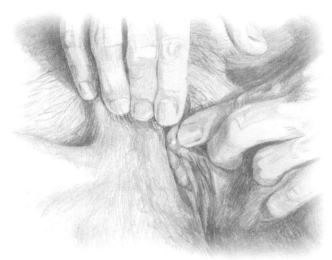

scenes in which he has sex with a woman who's pinned against a wall. Stroke upward from her introitus to the bottom of the clitoris, and pin the shaft and bottom of the clitoris against her body (FIGURE 2.4). This can feel exquisite to a woman, and you may notice some strong contractions. Report all sensations. If at any point, whether while stroking her or before, you feel your penis getting engorged, let her know that you feel her there. Tease her by asking her what "nasty thoughts" she's thinking. There is a very high correlation between your penis getting engorged and her thinking about it.

You can also tease your partner by playing with her clitoris through her hood. Slowly press your finger against the clitoral hood, adding more pressure if it feels good to do so. You might notice contractions and the engorgement of her clitoris as you do this (FIGURE 2.5).

TEASING WHILE DOING ✎ Teasing does not have to end once you begin stroking and peaking your partner (the "peaking" technique, an essential part of the EMO, is discussed in detail in later chapters). You can use teasing to take your partner higher than she thought she was ready to go. Sometimes, while I am doing someone, I tell her, "This is the last peak," or ask her if she has had enough—even when I know she still wants more. Some women hold out until the last peak and only then start to feel more. If she thinks that you will soon stop touching her, that often makes her get off better.

We have noticed that when a person deliberately asks for more, she opens herself up to feeling more. If the request for more does not feel genuine and enthusiastic, however, you are advised to stop unless your partner can generate enough enthusiasm to make you feel differently. But as long as she continues to feel more each time, you can keep saying, "This is going to be the last peak" after each previous "last peak." In some training sessions, we actually have quit stroking, removed the latex gloves that we wear during these sessions, and pretended that we were done, only to put on another pair of gloves and start bringing the student up again. This way, she is caught quite unaware, and her defenses are down. Sometimes this method has enabled a student to experience a number of additional peaks and to have the best orgasm of her life.

As we have said before, a woman may still resist even after she has gotten naked, lain down on the bed, and let you put your hand on her pussy. She might even resist feeling in her consciousness the orgasm that she is physically demonstrating. She can be engorged, having strong contractions, and showing all the signs of orgasm, all without being "at home" to these feelings.

These resistances can be viewed as an opportunity to play a game. They offer a reason for you, the doer, to be more enthusiastic, more confident, more communicative, and more playful. Enjoy the resistances, and continue with your seduction. You must be able to continually seduce the woman you are doing. This does not mean that you always will need to seduce her in the future, but you have to show a willingness and an ability to seduce. Only touch her when it is irresistible. You want her to want your touch. Tease her lightly over her genital area and over her pubic hair. The push/pull game, which we discussed earlier, continues into the do itself. Always notice whether she is going up or down, whether she's moving toward or away from you, and how strongly she is moving.

If you notice that she is mentally unaware of the orgasm her body is demonstrating, this means she is slowly going away from you. Point out the contractions and other signs, such as the fact that she is engorged, wet, and flushed. Have her put attention on her body rather than on her head, where

she is thinking and analyzing too much. Many people have a difficult time getting out of their heads and into the sensations of their pleasure centers. Make sure she pays attention to her pleasure. It is always safe to take a break and start up again later; this can help to increase her consciousness of her body's pleasurable sensations.

You can even play a game to find out what she can feel. Use anything from a feather to a slap on the clitoris, depending on the circumstances and your agreements with her beforehand. You can tug on her pubic hair, using a grasp anywhere on the spectrum from gentle to strong. You can play with ice, either by placing it directly on her genitals or by dripping it on her clitoris and other parts of her vulva. Ice can be used to tease a hot and throbbing penis, too. (Some people love ice, but some don't.) The idea is to play, have fun, and be curious.

Talk is by far your best weapon in overcoming her resistance. Whenever you point out something you notice happening in her body or something you feel in yours, she has an opportunity to go there with you and to put her attention on the pleasure. Telling her that you notice what she feels allows her to feel it more deeply. You can ask her to relax or to feel a specific spot or stroke. You can ask her to feel your finger. You can ask her to feel your thumb at the base of her introitus and to notice the contractions she has there. Then ask her to feel your finger on her clitoris. Let her know when her body responds positively to your requests. Give her a "win"—in other words, let her know she's succeeded at something. You also can ask her to take her sensation higher, to feel more—you are not saying that she doesn't feel enough already, but that you know she can go even higher. See "Ideas for Communication," at the back of the book, for more things you can say.

You must be willing to stop or at least take a break at a moment's notice. She may say something that causes you to feel negative. Such statements can be disguised pretty well, so she might say something that sounds good but feels lousy to you. For example, she may say she loves the circular stroke that you are using, when in reality it's an up-and-down stroke. If this happens, take a break, and point it out. You have to learn to trust your feelings, and you have to have the integrity to follow through on what your body tells you. Once you feel better, you can start again if you wish. Express your feelings!

Many women enjoy fantasy. You can stimulate your partner's imagination during a do with thoughts and words rather than actions. For example, you do not have to actually spank or whip her if those thoughts turn her on; simply introduce the idea into her head. Some women are turned on by the thought of having sex outdoors. We knew a woman who was turned on by thoughts of being in a jungle. She fantasized that her clitoris was a lioness on the hunt; it ran through the jungle and captured and devoured its prey. Another woman loved the thought of sex on a train, and another fantasized about doing it in outer space. When this latter woman's partner touched her, she imagined they were blasting into orbit. Each time the peaks grew higher, they passed a planet, until they were traveling past the stars at warp drive. She appreciated her partner's ability to notice when she went higher and to respond to that by providing visual images that enhanced her pleasure. It was important that he developed and exercised his sensitivity to her responses, his skill of paying close attention. If she had been resisting him at a certain moment, for example, and he'd chosen that moment to say that the rocket was blasting off, the imagery would have backfired, and the mission would have had to be scrubbed. In such a case, he could modify the flying metaphor by saying something such as "We are on the runway; the plane is picking up speed, about to take off—but now the captain has put on the brakes." This way, she would know his attention was on her and that he was right there with her. Then he could say that, this time, he will be the captain, and that he won't apply the brakes this time—she is going to take off without glitches. He could tease her by offering her the option of staying on the ground and passing on this orgasmic trip. Such are the fun games you can use to include imagination and conceptual thought in the mix of a do. Not all women or men want to play these games, and the games are unnecessary in order to have or produce an EMO. But they can be a fun addition to your bag of tricks, one you can use when appropriate.

Our goal is not to give you a formula that you can use every time out, rain or shine. As we have stated before, sometimes you want to go directly for the crotch and skip the teasing. Other times, you spend the majority of time teasing, touching only a little. Each experience is unique, so you do best to keep an open mind and to be ready to use whatever technique works. The more tools you have in your bag, the more prepared you are for any situation.

Same-Sex Relations: Some Observations

We have received mail from lesbian readers who agree with much of the sensual information we included in our first book and teach in our classes, and who report that they have practiced similar techniques for years.

A woman does not have to be a lesbian or even bisexual to enjoy rubbing or being rubbed by another woman. In fact, a second turned-on woman added to the combination of a woman and a man—even if the second woman just sits on the bed during the do—can cause the woman who's getting done to "give it up" more easily. (However, many people won't want to explore this option, although reportedly most men fantasize about being in bed with two women at one time.)

Why does a second woman add something to the mix? Women are less likely to fake their pleasure when another woman is close by, watching and feeling. It is more difficult for a woman doee to pull the wool over a man's eyes when another woman is present. In addition, a second woman can bring her own turn-on to the party. For this reason, whenever we engage in professional sessions with a female student, there is always at least one other woman in the room. In addition, we almost always demonstrate an EMO on a trained woman, in a new student's presence, before we do a new student herself. This allows the student not only to witness what she will experience but to feel the orgasm of the other woman and to allow it to jump-start her own orgasmic sensations. Women can turn on at will; they just require a reason to do so, and witnessing another woman's orgasm is often reason enough.

A woman who does another woman does not have to seduce her only with words and actions. She may also use her turn-on (a woman's ability to stimulate another with her desire and to create a physical response in that person—in this case the response is sexual excitement) to overcome her partner's resistance. Women are able to turn on other women as well as men, because women themselves are the source of turn-on and can direct it toward either sex. Women also can be turned on by another woman who is turned on, if they so choose. This is why seemingly turned-on women are used to sell everything from magazines to beer to cars. Almost everyone can respond to them.

Society may hold that men who experiment with giving and receiving pleasure from other men are gay. But, in fact, we know a number of straight men who have experimented with other men in a safe, non-threatening environment. The prejudice is so strong, however, that they usually experimented only with a woman present. Men cannot turn on at will, but they can tease and seduce each other, in the same way that they can seduce a woman.

Mail we have received from gay men indicates that they usually engage in sexual activity more frequently than heterosexual or lesbian couples. A man who knows how to produce an EMO often focuses a lot of attention on his partner. Men, whether gay or straight, are "success junkies"; by that token, they seem more likely than women to want to spend a great deal of time producing an orgasm in someone else's body. So not only are gay men more likely to have sex more frequently, but also they are more inclined to giving their partners more attention than most women would be when the men do have sex and know how to produce an EMO.

The teasing and seduction techniques we've discussed earlier in the book are as useful for gays and lesbians as they are for straight people—all these tactics help your partner to feel more. For people of any orientation, EMOs are about having more fun. EMOs are about noticing your partner and doing what it takes to cause them to feel their bodies and to intensely desire or crave to be touched and stimulated. There are no formulas to follow. You simply need to create and play with those techniques that seem most pleasurable and useful each time out. This is not difficult, as long as you focus close attention on your partner and yourself.

Lubricants

Friction is the force that resists motion as one thing rubs against another. When you touch someone for pleasure, possibly for an extended period of time, you want things to go smoothly; that means controlling the amount of physical friction that is produced as you rub. Lubricants applied to the hand of the person giving the orgasm or to the genitals of the person getting the orgasm reduce friction. Too much friction on your partner's genitals can cause pain and even abrasions. Too little friction and your hand slides all over the place. The selection of the right lubricant is vital to creating just the right amount of slipperiness. A number of lubricants are available, and each one has its benefits and its drawbacks. We recommend trying several to see what feels best to you and your partner.

CHOOSING A LUBRICANT There are many water-soluble lubricants on the market. You can find them in the personal-hygiene section of most drugstores, or on the Internet under "lubrications for sex." Some of their brand names are K-Y Jelly, Today, Astroglide, Foreplay, and Perform. One, called I-D Juicy Lube, comes in twelve flavors, from vanilla to piña colada. The viscosity, staying power, and taste of each lubricant differ; that is why it is best to check them out for yourself.

The benefits of water-soluble lubricants include the following: they are fun to apply; they won't stain the sheets or your clothes; you can easily wash them off your body; you can use them with latex; and putting them in your mouth is not too distasteful. The major drawback is that you have to keep reapplying them if you rub for an extended time, as they tend to get sticky after a while. You can add water to the lubricant if it starts to feel sticky; this reduces the stickiness and "freshens" the lubricant.

The other type of lubricant is the water-insoluble type. These are petroleum-derived and are also available in the drugstore. The best-known water-insoluble lubricant is Vaseline; in this case, the name brand is better than the generic alternatives. We have known people who adore Vaseline and will not use anything else, and many others who can't stand the feel of Vaseline and will use anything but. Another water-insoluble lubricant that we like is Albolene; it is actually a makeup remover and may be more difficult to find than Vaseline. Some people even use massage oils.

Benefits of water-insoluble lubricants include the following: they last for a long time once applied and therefore do not have to be reapplied, and they are probably better at protecting the skin than water-soluble options are. The drawbacks: they break down the latex in gloves or condoms, so they cannot be used with latex; it is difficult to remove the stains they produce from sheets; they are more difficult (although not impossible) to wash off the body; they taste pretty bad (you can add flavored oils); and they are less fun to apply, especially to a woman's genitals.

We use latex gloves when we work with students, so we use water-soluble lubricants when teaching, whether privately or in demonstrations. Likewise, we recommend that people use latex gloves (and therefore water-soluble lubricants) until they know their partners intimately. Although hand-to-genital contact is comparatively safe, a small open wound or cut could be present on any skin surface; gloves minimize the risk of communicating blood-borne sexually transmitted diseases.

Some people like to use their own saliva as a lubricant. If both partners are in agreement, they can choose whatever lubricant they like, including saliva. Saliva is like a water-soluble lubricant; it dries up quickly and has to be reapplied often. It tastes okay and it won't stain, but it can spread viral or bacterial infections in both directions. Some women are very prone to urinary-tract and genital infections; in such cases, saliva is not a good idea. Additionally, if you intend to give your partner a very intense and long ride, having to stop and keep reapplying saliva could prevent your partner from going as high as he or she might otherwise. On the other hand, saliva is a great lubricant if you plan to go back and forth between oral sex and manual stimulation.

Some of the water-soluble lubricants come with the spermicide nonoxynol-9 added. Nonoxynol-9 is a detergent, and it has been shown to

destroy some viruses, including the virus for HIV. However, used over an extended period of time, or even less, nonoxynol-9 has been shown to cause abrasions. Since HIV can gain entrance into the body through tears in the skin, this could defeat the purpose. Nonoxynol-9 also has caused abrasions and rashes on the hands of people who used it frequently, and it tastes bad to boot. We have not found any woman or man who likes the way it feels on their genitals. They all say it causes a burning or stinging sensation even after its removal.

Choose whatever lubricant you like best. You can make a fun game out of getting a number of different lubricants and testing each to see which ones feel the best and which ones you associate with the most intense orgasms. When you learn about a new product, check it out and compare it to your favorites. If you and your partner prefer different lubricants, keep them both around. Feel free to create any style and stroke to lubricate your partner. Different lubricants present new opportunities to craft original ways to apply them.

LUBRICATING A WOMAN ⟫ We like to use K-Y Jelly when we do a DEMO class. It spreads very easily, and we use a fun application stroke that is very pleasurable to the woman and looks great to the audience. Place a dab of lubricant about ½ inch in diameter on the last joints of your index and middle fingers (FIGURE 2.6), on the fingers' pad side.

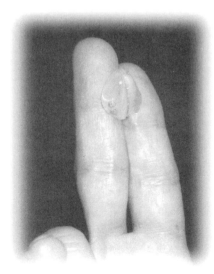

FIGURE 2.6
Putting a glob of lubricant on fingers for spreading on the vulva

Holding the two fingers together, apply the dab directly to the perineum of the doee, and slowly, with medium to light pressure, bring your fingers up her introitus. With this upward stroke, you lubricate her inner lips at the same time (FIGURE 2.7). As you reach the point directly beneath the clitoris, spread your fingers to avoid touching or lubricating it. Keeping the fingers spread, continue the upward movement so that each of the two

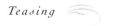

fingers finishes the stroke by lubricating the top area of the inner lips (FIGURE 2.8). By lubricating this way, you tease the clitoris. You single it out as the one area that remains untouched, unlubricated. As with other types of teasing, the woman, especially a trained one, may already be having contractions at this point.

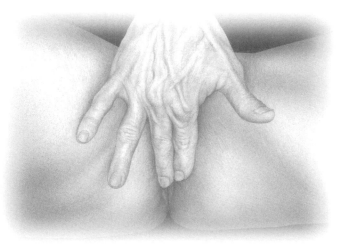

FIGURE 2.7
Application of water-soluble lubricant starting from the perineum with two fingers together

Also avoid lubricating the clitoral hood (see Chapter 3, "Genital Anatomy"); a slippery hood is tricky to anchor and pull up later. It is also important to keep the thumb of your doing hand lubricant-free, which makes retracting the hood less difficult.

After applying the lubricant, just stroke over the inner lips and introitus with one finger, going up toward the clitoris. Besides collecting any unused lubricant, this stroke is fun. You are actually spreading the lubricant to the area under the clitoris that you originally missed. (This also can be an opportunity to use the "Michael Douglas" stroke, described above.) A little trick I like is removing any excess lubricant and putting it

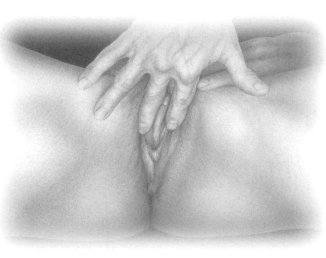

FIGURE 2.8
Spreading the fingers to avoid applying lubricant to the clitoris

FIGURE 2.9
Excess lubricant placed on back of hand as a "reservoir"

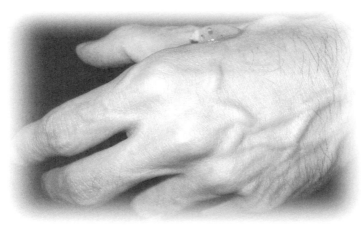

on the back of my hand to act as a reservoir. This allows me easy access to lubricant when I want to reapply it, so I don't have to pick up the tube again. Put the lubricant you collect on the back of your free hand between the thumb and index finger (FIGURE 2.9), or anywhere it won't get in the way.

If you're using Vaseline or Albolene, it works best to apply the lubricant to one small area at a time as you slowly approach the clitoris. You can tease the clitoris by lubricating every other part of the genitals first. Start with the perineum. Then get some more Vaseline or Albolene and lubricate one labia at a time. Slowly work your way toward the clitoris, but leave it dry until you are ready to stroke it.

Even after her genitals have been lubricated, you still do not have to go to her clitoris right away. You can continue to tease her with any of the teasing strokes described above. Any time you approach the clitoris and then back away, it's a tease. When you do finally decide to touch her spot, put a small amount of lubricant on the tip of your index or middle finger. Then pull back the clitoral hood as discussed in Chapter 3, "Genital Anatomy," hook your finger under the hood, and start stroking.

Sometimes a woman may have an irritation on her labia or her perineum, and it may not feel good to her to be touched at all on those areas. But her clitoris may be perfectly healthy, and she may like and want to be done. If this is the case, you can skip the lubrication of the labia and perineum. Avoid touching them, and touch her clitoris only with lubricant and with your fingers.

LUBRICATING A MAN   Water-soluble lubricants spread more easily on a penis than their water-insoluble counterparts. With a water-soluble lubricant, you can use a large amount at once and spread it easily over the entire penis. With a water-insoluble lubricant, by contrast, it works best to lubricate one side—or one part of a side—of the penis at a time, working your way up to the head and apex, or tip, the most sensitive part. Even with a water-soluble lubricant, you may want to take your time in lubricating the penis and do just one area at a time. You can leave the apex as the last area that you lubricate. This draws attention to it and is a way of teasing it. How you spread the lubricant depends on how much time you have and how much you like to tease.

Some people like to first warm the lubricant in their hands by rubbing their palms together—getting the hands all lubricated—before touching the penis. I prefer the lubricant, even if it's cold, to be directly applied to my penis. Once the penis is coated with lubricant, the hands easily glide along it. Some men enjoy cold lubricant and cold hands, and others like them warmed up. Find out what your man prefers, and act accordingly.

We have explored the use of teasing to take your partner higher and to bring him or her to a place of desire and willingness to surrender. We pick this theme up again—and go into more detail about peaking—in the chapters "Receiving an EMO," "Giving an EMO," and "Coming Down." First, however, we turn our attention to some essential basics on genital anatomy and masturbation.

CHAPTER THREE

Even though we may not remember our very young years, many of us enjoyed being played with and taught by our parents during that time. Those of us who are now parents ourselves have probably played games to teach our children about different aspects of life. One very common such game is the naming game. The mother or father points to a part of their body or the child's body and identifies it. Then the toddler is supposed to repeat the name of the body part. The parents point to the child's nose, mouth, ears, toes, or belly button—to every part of the anatomy except the genitals. No one we know ever got to name those mysterious parts, even though a lot of us were really curious about them. By not mentioning those "forbidden" areas, our parents conditioned us not to talk about them.

Genital Anatomy

As we grew up, we were still fascinated by those forbidden areas, but we were a little afraid to give them too much attention. Sometimes as boys and girls, we played "doctor" to investigate our own and our friends' "private" parts. If our parents found out about what we were doing, they most likely put the kibosh on such activities. We have heard countless stories from our students about how they were discovered playing in their garage or room by their parents, who threw a fit and forbade them to ever "do that" again.

When we are born—and even when in utero—we enter a world of sensation. The tactile sense is the first sense to develop in utero and probably is the most advanced of all our early senses. Although babies can't clearly distinguish among the senses, they can tell whether a sensation is more or less intense, and they express preferences early. They prefer being well fed to being hungry; they prefer being dry, clean, and warm to being wet, smelly, and cold. We know what we like and what we don't like, and from the very beginning we let our parents know how we feel about it.

As we develop and learn about the world and about how our body senses things—such as how light stimulates our eyes, how sound enters through our ears, how smells and tastes are sensed by our nose and mouth, and how we feel touch all over our skin, in some places more intensely than others—we are at the same time taught and conditioned to avoid those mysterious areas that also feel the best. We are trained never to touch them or talk about them. Vera's grandmother tucked Vera in at night, and if Vera's hands were below the covers, her grandmother made sure she placed them above the covers. Vera did not understand why her grandmother did this until years later.

Since most of us who grew up in this culture were not allowed to look at, touch, or learn about these pleasurable areas of our anatomy, it is not surprising how little most people know about their genitals and the genitals of the opposite sex. In this chapter we explore and illustrate the basic anatomy of both the female's and the male's "private" parts. We compare the differences as well as the similarities between them. Although every

person is different "down there," a common enough anatomy exists among most human beings that looking at pictures can help you locate and comprehend specific parts of the genitals.

Next time you are in bed with your partner, take a good look at each other's private parts. Make friends with them. The way you make friends is to get to know them better. Find out as much as you can about your partner's genitals; learn where it feels best to them to be touched, and learn how they like to be touched. (There are specific exercises in Chapter 8, "Pressures," that will help you each discover how you best like to be touched.) Discover what they smell, taste, and feel like, as well as what they look like.

According to science, the anatomy of male and female fetuses is the same for the first six weeks or so after conception. Between the sexes, only one out of forty-six chromosomes differs: males have an X and a Y chromosome, whereas females have two X chromosomes. A gene on the Y chromosome causes the development of the male fetus to proceed in a different direction from that of the female. The tissue and organs remain basically the same, but they are changed morphologically and spatially in the two sexes. We call these similar but different body parts *homologous*.

✑ Female Genital Anatomy ✑

Few people—male or female—have really investigated a woman's genitals. We have been conditioned to have sex in the dark, under the sheets. Even looking at a woman's genitals is considered taboo in many cultures. Many people in our society do not even have a name for the female genitals, calling them "down there," "mu mu," or other childish names. Some people even call the entire genital region the "vagina," even though the vulva is the more correct term—the vagina is the internal cavity, and the vulva is the external genitalia. In order to become an expert in giving a woman an EMO, you need to become familiar with the different parts and functions of her genitals. One initial piece of advice: It is a good idea to ensure there's good lighting in the room—this is necessary for this initial investigation as well as when giving her an EMO.

CLITORIS The *clitoris* (shown along with the vulva in FIGURE 3.1) is a most amazing organ. It means *key* in Greek, and it certainly is the key to unlocking a woman's pleasure. In fact, its only known function is to feel pleasure. The clitoral head has the highest concentration of pleasure nerve endings of any part of the male or female anatomy (eight thousand, according to Natalie Angier, in *Woman: An Intimate Geography*), yet it practically has been kept a secret to all but the really curious. Until the last couple of decades, very little information about the clitoris could be found in books or anywhere else. Physically, too, it is quite elusive and can remain hidden under its hood or prepuce (see below). It may remain hidden for a whole lifetime in some women who have never been stimulated.

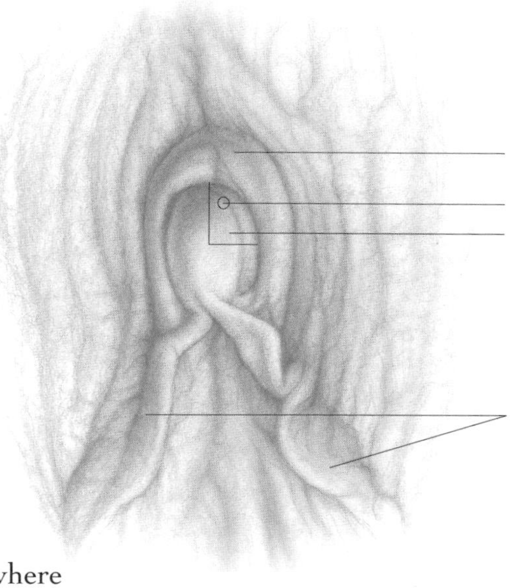

FIGURE 3.1
The vulva showing a large, engorged clitoris with a retracted hood

RETRACTED HOOD

1:30 SPOT

UPPER LEFT QUADRANT

LABIA MINORA

The clitoris is actually made up of three parts: the *glans*, the *shaft*, and the *crura*. The part that can become visible is the *head*, or glans (not to be confused with *glands*, which are tissues that secrete). The head can range in size from hardly visible (sometimes falsely called an "infantile clitoris") to a huge thumb-size appendage, although these extremes are rare. When stimulated, most engorge to at least two or three times their flaccid size, which is, on average, about a quarter-inch in diameter.

The shaft of the clitoris connects the glans to the crura, or *root*, of the clitoris, which is anchored in the pelvic cavity. The head is the most sensitive part of the clitoris, but the shaft and roots are both responsive to touch and can be pleasurably stimulated. You can feel the shaft through the skin where it disappears into the body. It is also possible to feel the shaft engorge with the proper stimulation. The crura of the clitoris is located inside the vagina, on the front of the vaginal wall; it is better known as the G-spot. You can read in detail about it in Chapter 9, "Insertion."

The clitoris is rather inconspicuous. It has been called "the little boy in the boat" by some of our old-timer friends. If you look at a woman's genitals without touching them, you are unable to see her clitoris or her vaginal opening. In most women the inner labia remain closed, the left and right lips touching each other. In most women the hood almost completely cov-

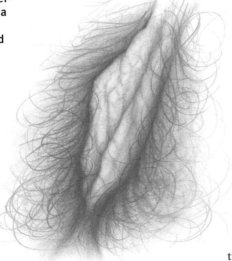

FIGURE 3.2
Female external genitalia with inner labia closed

ers the clitoris. Some women have a seemingly double- or even triple-layered hood, but it all moves neatly out of the way when desired. Depending on how much pubic hair she has, almost her entire genital region may be camouflaged. This entire area is a secret treasure that requires exploration (FIGURE 3.2).

In order to investigate further, you have to brush back the pubic hair, separate the labia, and pull back the clitoral hood. Some women have a lot of pubic hair and others have very little. Some women shave off all their pubic hair and others may shave up to a bikini line. You can use your hands to play with the pubic hair (as we discussed in the "Teasing" chapter, preceding this one). You can also use your hands to brush away the pubic hair from the clitoris and the inner labia so you can see what her genitals look like and what you will be touching. The hair may fall back into place, so you may have to push it aside more than once.

There are no known major diseases of the clitoris. A woman's vaginal area may become infected with a variety of diseases, and the labia and perineum may contract herpes sores, but we have never seen a clitoris with any such afflictions, and so it usually can be touched under most circumstances.

LABIA MINORA, LABIA MAJORA, AND INTROITUS The *labia minora,* or *inner labia* (lips), are quite sensitive to the touch. A woman has two inner labia, one on either side of her introitus (the vaginal opening). They are made of erectile tissue and become engorged with blood when a woman is stimulated. They come in a variety of shapes and sizes. We have seen some that barely extended from the woman's body and others so huge they looked like two large ears protruding from her genitals. Most inner labia fall some-where between these two extremes. The labia minora often extend upward and connect to the clitoris or clitoral hood, or both, on each side.

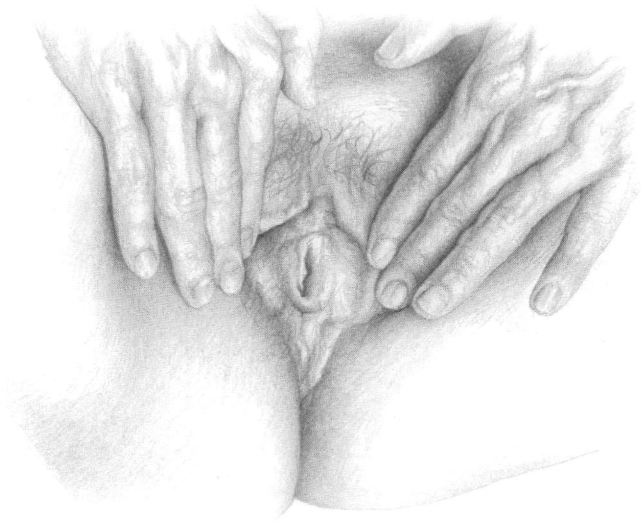

FIGURE 3.3
Separation of inner labia exposing the vaginal opening

You can separate the inner labia by plac-ing your hands on either side of the inner labia—that is, on the outer labia—and pulling them gently apart. You can do this with your thumbs or with all your fingers and your palms (FIGURE 3.3). They separate easily whichever way you do it. Once the labia are separated, they usually stay that way for the duration of the sex act.

When you separate the labia, you expose the *vaginal opening,* or *introitus.* This is composed of very shiny mucous tissue. When a woman is turned on, you may notice some lubrication or wetness here. You also can see her *uri-nary* or *urethral opening,* which is a small slit between the vaginal opening and the clitoral area.

The area just outside the inner labia is called, conveniently, the *outer labia,* or *labia majora. Labia* is Latin for *lips,* and the inner labia are very liplike, in both texture and appearance. The outer labia appear less like lips and more like mounds. Pubic hair often grows on them, while the inner labia are usually hairless. The outer labia may also engorge with genital arousal.

CLITORAL HOOD ❦ Hoods are loose, protective coverings. They keep the rain off our heads and the backs of our necks; on an automobile, a hood covers the engine. (*Hood* is also slang for *hoodlum* or short for *neighborhood*, but neither of those meanings concern us here.)

The *hood*, or *prepuce*, of the clitoris is what we are concerned with (FIGURE 3.4). It protects the clitoris from external abrasion. This cover is usually, but not always, loose. Clitoral hoods come in all types, from very loose-fitting to so snug that they are difficult or even impossible to retract. We have seen more than one woman whose hood was attached to her clitoris from top to bottom. Other clitorises seem to be covered by a multilayered hood.

You can touch the clitoris either directly or through the hood. Many women believe they are too sensitive to be touched directly on the head of their clitorises, so they masturbate and direct their lovers to touch them through their hoods. In our experience, of the dozens of women who have reported this supersensitivity, we have not yet found one who could not be directly touched on the head of her clitoris when proper lubrication and knowledgeable techniques were applied.

You can pleasurably stimulate a woman and even produce an EMO by touching her clitoris through the hood. It is fun to tease a woman by

FIGURE 3.4
Outer female genitalia showing the hood covering the clitoris

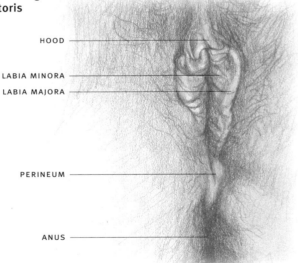

HOOD

LABIA MINORA

LABIA MAJORA

PERINEUM

ANUS

deliberately touching her spot—located on the upper left quadrant (from the woman's perspective) of the clitoris in most women—and other parts of her clitoris in this indirect manner. (See FIGURE 2.5 in the "Teasing" chapter.)

For women whose hoods don't retract, touching the clitoris through the hood is the best and most effective way to produce an EMO. For all other women, at least in our experience, the best and most effective way to create an EMO is by pulling back the hood— moving it out of the way—and putting a finger directly on the exposed, naked clitoris. There are a number of ways to pull back the hood; we describe and illustrate some of these techniques below.

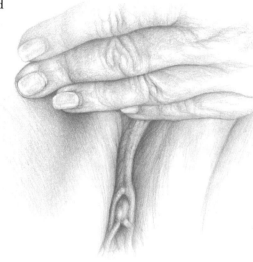

FIGURE 3.5
A woman retracting the hood from her own clitoris with her palm

When masturbating, a woman can pull back her own hood by placing the palm of her second hand—the one that will not be doing the stroking— upon her pubic area, just over the hood and clitoris, pressing the hand into her body, and pulling upward (FIGURE 3.5). She can also use a couple of fingers of her free hand to pull back the hood (FIGURE 3.6)

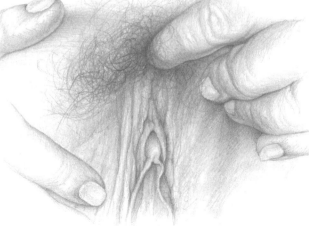

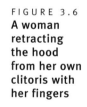

FIGURE 3.6
A woman retracting the hood from her own clitoris with her fingers

If you're right-handed, the best way to pull back the hood when you are doing a woman is to place the thumb of your right hand against the left side (from the woman's perspective) of the hood and clitoris and pull upward on the hood while pressing against the clitoris and clitoral shaft. You do not want to press too roughly against the clitoris, as that may hurt her, but press firmly enough that the hood moves out of the way (FIGURE 3.7). You may be unable to retract the hood off the entire clitoral head, but pull it up as far as you can. Next, place the index or middle finger of your right hand under the hood and onto her spot. You should be able to see that you are at the right location. Keep your thumb firmly against the left side of the clitoral shaft while you stroke the head of her clitoris. The more engorged her clitoris gets, the more it will be exposed and visible and will move away from the hood.

Left-handed doers actually have a slight advantage over right-handed ones, because when they pull back the hood with the thumb, their index and middle fingers are at the perfect angle to reach her spot. The best way for a left-handed person to retract the hood is to place the left thumb against the right side of the clitoris and hood and press inward and upward as much as possible. The hood of the clitoris should move up and out of the way, exposing the head of the clitoris (FIGURE 3.8). A firm, confident touch is appropriate here, and it is always a good idea to communicate—especially at first—to find the pressure that feels best.

Some people have a difficult time retracting the hood with the thumb. But this is a really important skill that one must master if one wishes to be a top-notch doer. We have heard all kinds of excuses for why people can't do

FIGURE 3.7
Pulling back the hood with thumb (right) to expose the clitoris

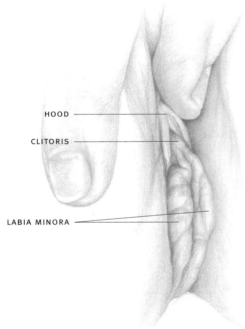

HOOD

CLITORIS

LABIA MINORA

this technique. We suggest practicing till you get it right. Let the woman you are doing know what you are up to. You may not want to practice for too long, as she may want you to get to her clitoris already. If such is the case, there are a couple of other ways to retract the hood, described below. Then, after she has gotten off, maybe she'll let you practice more, or maybe you can bring her down while your thumb practices the retraction technique described above.

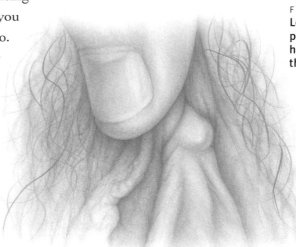

FIGURE 3.8
Left thumb pulling up on hood to expose the clitoris

Each time you do her, you can spend some time perfecting this technique for your bag of tricks.

An easier way to pull back the hood is to place the palm of your non-doing hand flat against the pubic area, right above the clitoris; now press inward and pull upward. This is very similar to the way a woman pulls back her own hood for masturbation, as described above. This technique does retract the hood, but it leaves your nondoing hand unavailable for other uses, such as insertion and feeling contractions. It also doesn't permit you to anchor the clitoris against the shaft, or to pinch the clitoris between your finger and thumb. The clitoris has a better chance of escaping your finger when it remains unanchored.

Another way to retract the clitoral hood is to get a good grip on a bunch of pubic hair above the clitoral area and then pull it upward and away from the clitoris. Avoid pulling only a few hairs at once, because that would hurt. Take a rather large handful. You can also ask the woman herself to pull back on her pubic area or pubic hair. Once the woman has been stroked for a while, her clitoris engorges and protrudes from the hood. When this occurs either you or she can let go of this grip.

In the "Insertion" chapter, we describe another way to pull back the hood, which involves inserting fingers into the vagina. But because we don't usually recommend such insertion at the beginning of a do, this technique is best used after the orgasm has been going on for a while.

PERINEUM The *perineum* is the area between the vagina and the anus. We had an old friend who said that when he was growing up they called this area the "taint." It ain't the vagina and it ain't the a-hole. (Men also have a perineum, which is the area between the anus and the scrotum; it is discussed later in the chapter.) This area can be played with and touched when teasing. A good number of nerve endings innervate it, and it can feel quite pleasurable when stimulated. Some women report really enjoying having their perineums stroked, and other women are indifferent. It is best to use lubricant when stroking here for any length of time.

When women give birth, doctors often perform an episiotomy, a procedure that cuts into the perineum to expand the opening of the vagina. This may be necessary in some instances, but it is probably performed more often than it has to be. A few of our students have endured poorly performed episiotomies; they had difficulty healing properly and experienced pain when touched in that area.

MONS PUBIS The *mons pubis*—also known as *mons veneris, mount of Venus*, or just *mons*—is the pad of fatty tissue and thick skin that covers the lowest area of a woman's abdomen. It lies in the triangular area between the upper part of her thighs, just above the vulva. Just below the mons pubis is the area of the pelvis where the pubic bones join. After puberty, the mons pubis is covered with pubic hair in most girls.

Men have a similar fatty pad above their genitals, although it is usually not as apparent as in women, especially if the man is on the slim side. This area can be pleasurably stimulated; the technique for doing so is described in the "Insertion" chapter.

➶ Male Genital Anatomy ➴

Women are typically more familiar with men's genitalia than the other way around. The penis and scrotum, since they're "outies," as opposed to women's "innies," are more visible, and penises are generally much more publicly acknowledged than clitorises are. Yet how many women have actually taken the time and effort to explore these organs? Male genitals, like female genitals, come in many different sizes and shapes.

PENIS ➶ The *penis* is a "multi-tool," as our friend Regena Thomashauer likes to call it. It not only is used for pleasure but serves as a urinating device and a seed-planting tool. Penises vary in size, both among individuals and even within an individual. The flaccid penis can range in size from hardly visible, when its owner is cold or frightened, to almost the size of an erect one in men with a low coefficient of expansion (in other words, whose penises don't grow much in erection). The largest erect penis reported was more than fourteen inches long. The average flaccid penis is around three inches long and $1\frac{1}{4}$ inch in diameter, and the average erect penis is a little longer than five inches and about $1\frac{2}{3}$ inches in diameter. The size and shape of an erect penis may also vary according to the sexual partner with whom it's engaged.

An erection is the result of blood flowing into the three parallel chambers of the flaccid penis. The amount of blood present in an erection is eight to ten times that present in the flaccid state. A baby is able to have an erection. Healthy men are able to get erections well into their eighties, although they may not be quite as hard or happen as often as when the men were younger. Most men experience nocturnal erections three to five times each night. These are not necessarily the result of sexual dreams but function to keep the penile tissue healthy.

The penis consists of nerves, blood vessels, fibrous tissue, and three parallel cylinders of spongy tissue. The bottom of the penis extends internally into the pelvic cavity. This part, including its attachment to the pubic bones, is referred to as the *root* of the penis. The external, visible portion of the penis,

FIGURE 3.9
Male anatomy

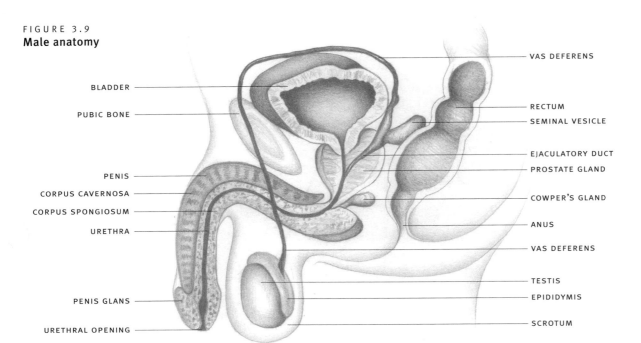

excluding the head, is known as the *shaft*. The shaft continues into the body and together with the root forms what we call the "hidden cock." The smooth, rounded-shaped head is called the *glans*.

The spongy tissue consists of the *cavernous bodies* and the *spongy body*. The two cavernous bodies *(corpora cavernosa)* lie side by side above the smaller third cylinder, the spongy body *(corpus spongiosum)*, which forms the glans, or head, at its extreme end (FIGURE 3.9). The cavernous and spongy bodies consist of spongelike irregular spaces and cavities. Each chamber is richly supplied with blood vessels. When a male is sexually excited, these chambers become engorged with blood. Numerous veins and capillaries are visible on an erect penis.

The spongy body also surrounds the *urethra,* which runs through it to the tip of the penis, where an opening, or *meatus,* allows urine and semen to exit. At the root of the penis, the innermost tips, or *crura,* of the cavernous bodies are connected to the pubic bones.

As you can see, the penis has three parts that bear the same names as the three parts of the clitoris: the glans, the shaft, and the crura. The head or glans of the penis, including the *apex*, or *frenulum*, is considered homologous to the clitoris, and the shaft of the penis is homologous to the inner labia.

FORESKIN ⤳ The penis comes in two distinct varieties, circumcised and uncircumcised, both of which have an equal capacity for getting erect. The difference between the two is that the *foreskin* has been removed in circumcised penises.

In an uncircumcised penis (FIGURE 3.10), the foreskin, or *prepuce,* is homologous to the hood of the clitoris. In newborns it is attached to the glans or head of the penis. As the child matures, this connection is broken, and the foreskin can be retracted to the bottom portion of the shaft. The ability to retract the foreskin usually develops in the first few years of life but occasionally occurs in puberty. The head of the penis is quite sensitive in the newborn; the purpose of the foreskin is to protect it from any kind of abrasion. "Infant smegma" basically consists of the dead skin cells that get caught under the foreskin. One only has to regularly wash the baby with soap and water to keep this area clean. At puberty, the *Tyson's gland,* located in the glans or head of the penis, starts secreting an oily substance that, when mixed with skin cells, produces "adult smegma." Again, soap and water easily takes care of this problem.

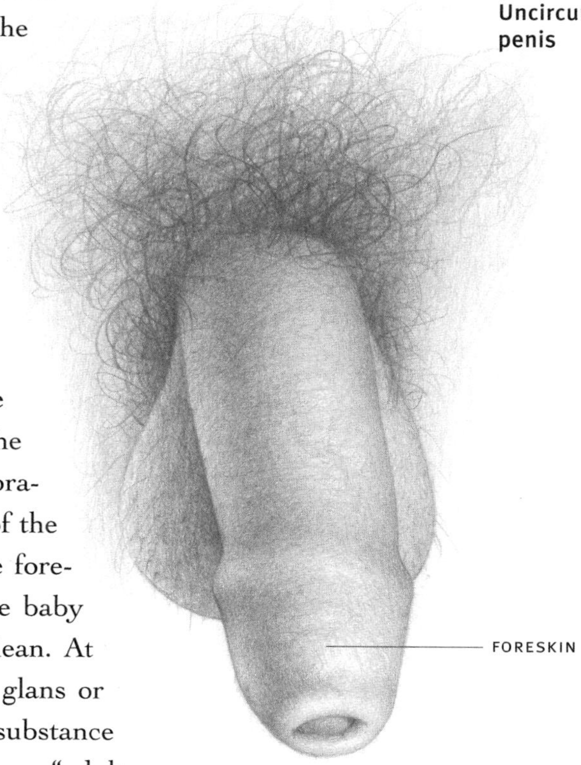

The foreskin of an uncircumcised man must be pulled back by the doer so that she can get her hand around the shaft and head of his penis.

FIGURE 3.10
Uncircumcised penis

FORESKIN

FIGURE 3.11
**Underside of
penis showing
the apex**

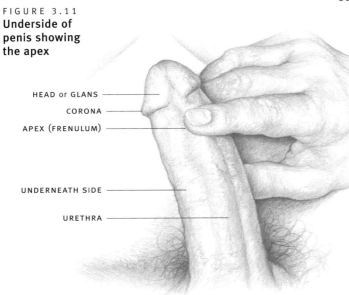

HEAD or GLANS

CORONA

APEX (FRENULUM)

UNDERNEATH SIDE

URETHRA

To pull back the foreskin, make a ring or semi-ring with the index finger and thumb of your nondoing hand. Place it around the penis and foreskin and pull back on the foreskin, toward the base of the penis. Once he engorges, the foreskin should remain retracted.

The circumcised penis is the same as the uncircumcised one, lacking only the foreskin. They both have a head and a shaft, which are separated by the *sulcus,* or *corona.* The area on the penis's underside, just below the corona, is called the *apex,* or *frenulum* (FIGURE 3.11). Also on the shaft's underside is the urethra, running along its middle. (By "underside," we mean the side of the shaft that rests against the scrotum when the penis is not erect; this more or less becomes the "top side" of the penis when it is erect. You can clearly see the underside in FIGURE 3.11.) The apex is the most sensitive area on most men's penises. The head of the penis also has a lot of nerve endings and is very sensitive.

SCROTUM, TESTES, AND PROSTATE The *scrotum,* or *scrotal sac,* contains the *testes* (see FIGURE 3.9, earlier). The scrotal sac is homologous to the labia majora on a woman. The testes are homologous to a woman's ovaries. The scrotum is a loose pouch of skin hanging from the abdominal wall directly underneath the penis. Normally it hangs loosely from the body wall, although it may shrivel and tighten toward the body due to cold temperatures or sexual arousal. The sac consists of two layers. The outer layer is thin skin that is darker in color than the skin of the rest of the body. It usually becomes sparsely covered with hair at puberty. The inner layer is the *tunica dartos,* made of muscle and connective tissue; it contracts to pull the testicles closer to the body when chilled or aroused. The sac is divided into two separate sections, one left and one right, each of which contains one *testi,* or *testicle.* Each testi is suspended by a *spermatic cord.* The spermatic cord houses the *vas deferens* (see below), nerves, *cremasteric muscle fibers,* and blood vessels. Sudden fear may cause strong contractions of the cremasteric muscle, pulling the scrotum closer to the body. One testicle (the left) usually hangs lower than the other.

The testes' two functions are to produce sperm and to secrete sex hormones, or *testosterone.* The testes usually migrate from inside the abdomen into the scrotum before birth. For optimal sperm production, the temperature of the testes is about three to five degrees cooler than the temperature of the rest of the body. Sperm are produced in the *seminiferous tubules* after puberty; these highly coiled tubes form the bulk of the testes. *Interstitial cells* are found between these tubules; they produce and secrete sex hormones directly into the bloodstream. The sperm from the tubules move into the *epididymis,* which are located in the top of each testi (again, see FIGURE 3.9). Here they are stored and mature.

From here, the sperm drain into the *vas deferens,* inside the spermatic cord. The vas deferens is a thin duct close to the scrotal surface. (This is the location where a vasectomy, the surgical procedure to induce sterilization in males, is easily performed.) The vas deferens enters the body and is joined by the excretory duct of the *seminal vesicles.* Together they form the *ejaculatory duct.* The seminal vesicles secrete an alkaline fluid high in fructose. This secretion makes up about two-thirds of the seminal fluid. Once combined with this secretion, the sperm are energized and can propel themselves with their tails.

A healthy *prostate* is about the size of a chestnut. It is typically pyramid-shaped, with its base attached to the bottom of the bladder. Its dimensions are approximately one inch by one and one-half inch by two inches. Both ejaculatory ducts, one from each testi, and the urethra pass through the prostate. The prostate secretes most of the rest of the seminal fluid—a thin, milky alkaline fluid that neutralizes the acid environment of the vagina—which combines with the secretions from the seminal vesicles and the sperm; then it all flows into the urethra. The prostate can be very pleasurably stimulated. Check the "Insertion" chapter.

The *Cowper's glands,* or *bulbourethral glands,* are small, lentil-size organs located right below the prostate on either side of the urethra (see FIGURE 3.9) They secrete a clear, slippery mucous fluid upon sexual arousal. This fluid may appear as small droplets at the tip of the glans before ejaculation. We have heard it called "glad come" by some of our older students. This secretion is not the same as semen; its probable function is to lubricate the urethra for seminal fluid passage. It does occasionally contain sperm; this is one of the reasons why the withdrawal method of birth control is risky.

EJACULATION ⟳ *Ejaculation* and orgasm are not the same. Men can experience orgasm without ejaculation. In men, orgasm can begin with or even before the first touch or stroke, just as in women. Ejaculation occurs when neural excitation surpasses a critical threshold. This usually happens in response to a physical stimulation, but "wet dreams" can occur with only a mental stimulus. One can also ejaculate without an engorged penis, although this is unusual.

Ejaculation occurs in two stages. The first is the emission stage, when the seminal fluid, including the sperm, flows into the urethral bulb. The prostate, seminal vesicles, and vas deferens all contract. The two urethral sphincters (internal and external) contract, which keeps the seminal fluid in the urethral bulb. This expansion of the urethral bulb gives a man a sense that ejaculation is forthcoming.

The second stage is the expulsion stage. The semen trapped in the urethral bulb is released as the external urethral sphincter relaxes. Strong rhythmic contractions occur in the muscles surrounding the bulb and the root of the penis. Contractions continue along the entire urethral passage. Once ejaculation is over—in less than ten seconds—and engorgement eases, the internal sphincter relaxes and urine can once again enter the urethra.

PERINEUM   Males, like females, have a *perineum*, the area between the bottom of the scrotum and the anus. This area can feel a lot of pleasure when stimulated properly. The prostate and "hidden cock" can be externally stimulated here. When you press under the scrotum to prevent ejaculation (we discuss this technique later in the book, in the chapters on how to give and receive EMOs), you prevent the seminal fluid from escaping all at once out of the urethral bulb. This may result in a slow seepage of semen and in a prolongation of the orgasm's intense state.

A knowledge of the anatomy, function, and capabilities of both men's and women's genitals will enable you to continue your quest to becoming a better sexer. You need not remember the names of all the parts we have just discussed, but having a general understanding of how things work and how they look will only aid you in giving your partner pleasure. The more you visually study your partner's pleasure centers, the better prepared you are to masterfully give your partner EMOs.

Now that you have studied the anatomies of the male and female genital area, we are perfectly positioned to continue to our next chapter, which deals with the best body and hand positions to produce the optimum orgasm in both women and men.

CHAPTER FOUR

In real estate they say, "Location, location, location. Everything has to do with location." In making an EMO, location may not be everything, but without a good location, one cannot expect to create a great orgasm. The word location here refers to the relative positions of the bodies of the people giving and receiving the orgasm. It also refers to positioning the hands so that they're most advantageously situated to stimulate each other's genitals, and it refers to the best angles from which to stimulate the clitoris, too. In this chapter, we explore the various body and hand positions that work best when creating the optimum orgasm.

Positions

Setting Up the Space

Setting up the space for the "do" (see FIGURE 4.1) is vitally important to creating an atmosphere of attention and readiness. The doer's goal is that the doee surrender his or her nervous system into the doer's hands. By arranging the space with care, the doer demonstrates his or her willingness to take control of the do, and that makes surrender likelier. It is good to set out pillows, towels, lubricant, and drinks (and even music and candles, if you want them) before starting so that one partner need not get up in the middle of the do to look for an item. You're setting the mood for pleasure, and the more pleasurable control of the space you can take, the more likely that the doee will give up resistance and surrender. If you can provide something special that the doee likes (such as a particular piece of music or a glass of fruit juice), that, too, shows your interest and attention and allows for more fun.

Now, on to the initial positions of both partners. Finding the best position is of the utmost importance if you are serious about pleasure, and this is especially true for the doer. In a good doing position, you have great manual access to your partner's genitals. Most of the positions demonstrated here allow you visual access as well. Having visual contact with the vulva or the penis is very beneficial when learning how to do—and how to put the greatest possible amount of attention on your partner. Most of the positions we recommend below also enable you to have some face-to-face access with your partner. This makes communication more clear and easier. The doer should find the most comfortable

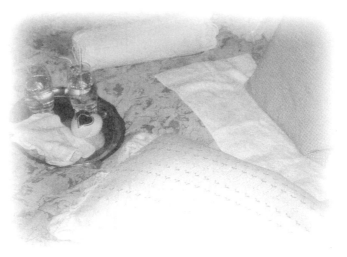

FIGURE 4.1
Setting up the space for the sitting position

position possible. You will "do" best if your body is relaxed except for the movements of your hands, eyes, and mouth. It is a good idea for the doer to use pillows to help him or her stay comfortably in one position for an extended amount of time. On the other hand, it is also okay for the doer to change positions once the do has begun. The uppermost goal is fun, and if it seems like fun to change your position, go ahead.

As the doee, you increase your chances for receiving the most pleasure if you are in a relaxed state. This means exerting as little energy as possible to sustain your position. Usually, your entire body should rest on a comfortable surface, such as a bed. A good mattress can only make the experience better. Most people spend several thousand dollars on a car, but only a fraction of that on a mattress, even though they spend much more time on the mattress. Ask yourself how important pleasure is to you. Pillows are helpful, too, and in this chapter we describe the proper placement of pillows for various positions. (Vera and I have twelve pillows of all shapes and sizes on our bed.)

When a woman is being done, she should spread her legs as wide apart as is comfortable and possible. This allows her partner optimal manual and visual access. Lots of men and plenty of women think they need to move their bodies and thrust their hips to help the orgasm along. However, when you're getting done, the best thing you can do is not move at all. Lie as still and relaxed as possible. Give your partner full control of your body. The more you move, the less control your partner has; moreover, if a woman thrusts about, it is hard for her partner to keep his hands on her clitoris.

Positions for Doing a Woman

THE SITTING POSITION   The position we use most often—our first choice—is one we call the "primo" or "sitting" position. (Before trying it, prepare the space with the necessary pillows, drinks, lubricant, and towels; see FIGURE 4.1, earlier.) The person giving the orgasm sits with his back against pillows at the head of the bed; preferably the pillows are braced against a wall or headboard. The woman getting done lies perpendicular to the doer. Her head is to the doer's right if the doer is right-handed (FIGURE 4.2) or to the doer's left if the doer is left-handed (FIGURE 4.3). Her legs are spread apart, and her outside leg is supported by a pillow. The doer's leg that corresponds to his dominant hand (right leg for a right-handed doer, left leg for a left-handed doer) is placed over the woman's abdomen, and his other leg is placed under her legs. Placing the doer's leg over the doee's abdomen allows him to rest the elbow or forearm of his "doing" hand on it. This is important because it prevents his arm from growing tired; if his arm grows tired, the doer's energy and attention is on his arm, not on the orgasm. His second hand is free to move around or to place under the woman's buttocks, with his thumb against her introitus.

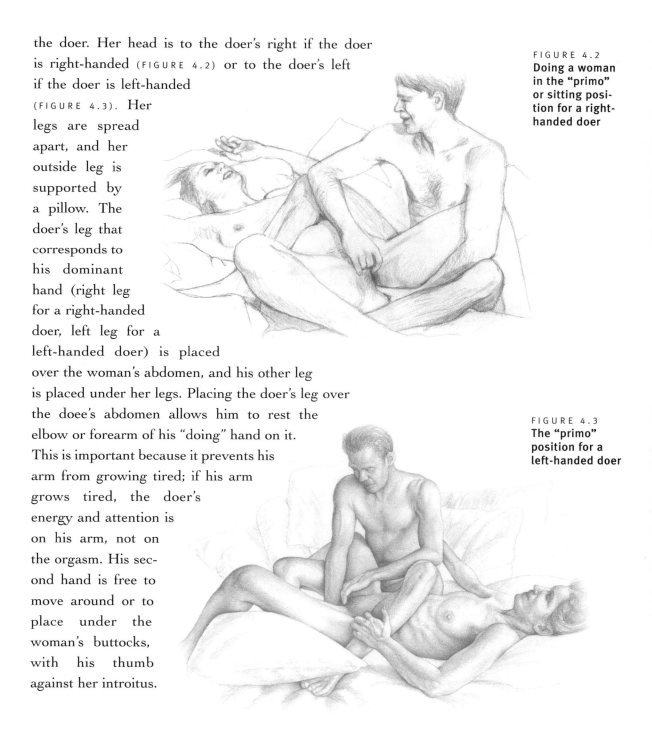

FIGURE 4.2
Doing a woman in the "primo" or sitting position for a right-handed doer

FIGURE 4.3
The "primo" position for a left-handed doer

The sitting position gives you maximum manual access to your partner's genitals, as well as a clear view of them. You also are in a great position to see her face and easily talk to her. Make sure that your shoulder is relaxed and your entire body is free of tension.

In a variation on the sitting position, the doer sits cross-legged instead of extending his legs over and under the doee. This position is a little less intimate, as you don't have your legs around your partner. It also requires the ability to sit cross-legged for an extended amount of time, which some people might find challenging. And since this position doesn't let you rest your elbow on your leg, we suggest putting a pillow over her abdomen and resting your elbow on that. You can place her inside leg over yours, or not, as you choose.

A second variation is the "chair" position. Your partner lies along the edge of the bed or on a couch. Her head should be on the same side as your doing hand. Pull a stool or chair up to the bed or couch so you can sit facing her. This position is even more formal; the doer can remain fully clothed if that feels best. By keeping your clothes on, you are communicating that you are there only to put attention on your partner; you won't seek reciprocation.

FIGURE 4.4
Doing a woman with the right hand on the clitoris while she is on a massage table and the doer is seated on a chair

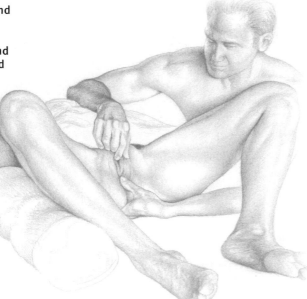

You may want to put a pillow on her abdomen so that you can lean over and rest your arm there.

We use a variation of the chair position in our DEMO class. The woman lies on a massage or gynecological table, with pillows placed under her thighs for support, and the doer sits on a chair perpendicular to her. If the doer is right-handed, he or she sits on her left; if the doer is left-handed, he or she sits on her right. The doer is able to talk to her or to swivel and talk to the class. His or her hands are right at the doee's genitals, and the doer has great visual access to them as well. The doer can rest the doing arm on her abdomen. (If you have bony elbows, like I have, you can place a pillow under your arm.) The second hand starts under the doee's inside leg, with the thumb resting at the introitus. Then, whenever the doer uses the fingers of the second hand to stimulate different areas of the vagina, the doer places the second arm over the doee's inside leg (FIGURE 4.4).

LYING ON YOUR SIDE ⋘ This is a good position, especially for a doer with an injured back. As the doer, you lie on your nondoing-hand side, with your head at the opposite end of the bed from your partner's head. Her legs are spread apart. Put a pillow under her outer thigh (the one farthest from you) and one over her inner thigh (the one closest to you). Lay your chest on the pillow that is over her inner thigh. Place your bottom (non-doing) hand between her legs, resting the forearm on the bed, with your thumb at her introitus and your fingers under her buttocks. Your doing-hand arm can rest on a small pillow on her abdomen, so your hand is free to stroke her genitals. You may want to use more pillows to support your back and your neck. In this position, you have great visual access to her genitals, but no direct facial contact. The position also allows only limited use of the second hand (FIGURE 4.5).

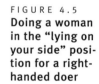

FIGURE 4.5
Doing a woman in the "lying on your side" position for a right-handed doer

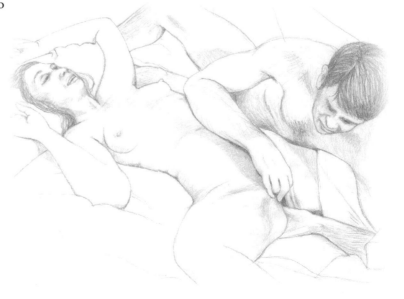

SIDE BY SIDE ☞ Here's a position that is fun—but not recommended for the beginner. The woman lies on the bed quite normally, with her head at the head of the bed and her legs spread apart. Her outer leg rests on a pillow. The doer lies parallel to her, on her right or left side. I am right-handed, so I prefer to be on her right side. This allows me to snuggle up to her, lie partially on my left side, and do her with my right hand. I place my left hand under her buttocks and play with her introitus and vagina. This is a wonderful position because it allows talking and kissing. You also are near her breasts, and she may want you to touch her there. It is best to know beforehand how and where she likes to be touched on her breasts. Generally, women like to be touched on the breasts more lightly than most men think they do. Some women may like their nipples squeezed, but this is usually after they have been clitorally stimulated for a while.

The drawback of this position is that you are unable to look at her genitals to see what you are doing. Anchoring the clitoral hood with your thumb is also more difficult in this position, and maneuverability of the bottom hand is hindered. This is not the best position from which to go for the most intense orgasm, but the close facial contact can greatly enhance intimacy. It is a nice position in which to wake up or go to sleep. It is very similar to the side-by-side position for coming together that we describe and illustrate later in the chapter (see FIGURE 4.12)

⟋ Positions for Doing a Man ⟍

BETWEEN HIS LEGS ☞ This is a good position in which the doer sits between the man's legs. Have him lie on a bed or any comfortable surface, with his legs spread wide enough apart for you to sit between them and facing him. Sit cross-legged or whatever way is comfortable for you. You can put his legs over or under yours (see FIGURE 4.6). Use pillows to support your back and other parts of your body. In this position, you are free to use both hands on his penis and/or scrotal area. You have an excellent view of what you are doing, and you can see his face for direct communication.

You can also bend over to place
his penis in your mouth if you are
so inclined.

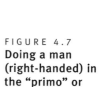

FIGURE 4.6
**Doing a man
while sitting
between his legs**

THE SITTING POSITION ⋙

The "primo" position that we
described above for doing a
woman is also excellent for
doing a man. The doer sits
against pillowed sup-
port, and the man lies
perpendicular to the doer.
If the doer is right-handed,
the man should lie with his head on the
doer's right side; if the doer is left-handed, he should lie with his head to the
doer's left. The doer places the leg that is on the same side as her doing hand
over the man's abdomen (right leg for a right-handed doer, left leg for a left-
handed doer) and the other leg under his legs. Both of the doer's hands are
free to manipulate his genital area (FIGURE 4.7), and the position allows good
visual contact with his genitals and face. The leg over his abdomen keeps
the man from thrusting and keeps him grounded. The doer can rest
her doing arm on her own upper leg, but this is less important than when you're doing a woman, as the doer's
movements in this position are less delicate.

FIGURE 4.7
**Doing a man
(right-handed) in
the "primo" or
sitting position**

In a variation, the doer can place her
bottom leg near the doee's penis
instead of under his legs.
The doer can then use the
foot and heel of this leg to
press against his "hidden
cock" area (see Chapter 3,
"Genital Anatomy").

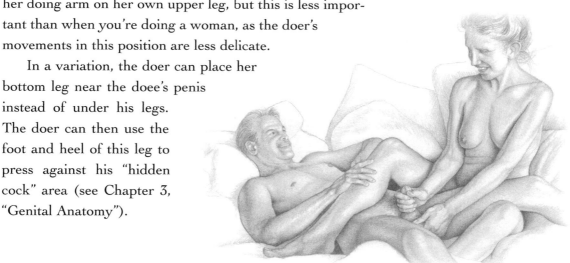

STRADDLING HIS LEG ❧ In this position, the doer lies at an angle at the man's side, so that she can straddle his leg between her own. The doer's head faces in the same direction as the man's head but is a little lower—about level with his upper arm, depending on the two people's relative heights. The doer has control, and she is also allowed direct pleasure via the contact of her genitals against his leg. The doer is also free to use her top leg or knee to play with his scrotal area or penis. This position can be executed from the right or left side; the drawback is that it allows good use of only one hand (FIGURE 4.8).

LYING ON YOUR SIDE ❧ You can also do a man while lying on your side with your head facing in the opposite direction from his. Place a pillow over his thigh if this feels comfortable and lay the side of your torso against it. Pillows can be used to make both parties more comfortable, so use them if desired. If you are left-handed, lie on your right side, and vice versa. Rest your bottom, non-doing hand between his legs. Your doing hand is free to play with his entire genital area. Your bottom hand is allowed only limited movement, but you have a great view of his genitals. This position also permits great access for cock sucking (FIGURE 4.9). Use as many pillows as you need to remain comfortable and to use your energy for feeling the pleasure and giving the orgasm.

FIGURE 4.8
Doing a man while straddling his leg

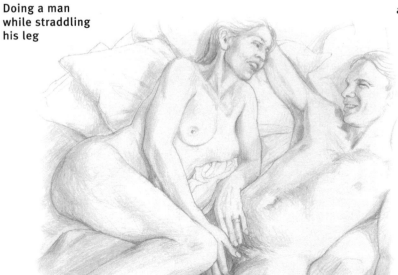

SIDE BY SIDE ❧ Another position for doing a man—as when doing a woman—is lying next to him in bed; both of your heads should face in the same direction. The doer lies slightly on her

side to allow her to reach over and play
with the doee's penis and genital area.
There is no visual access to the
genitals, but the face-to-
face contact allows
great intimacy. Again,
this is similar to the
side-by-side "coming
together" position, below
(see FIGURE 4.12).

ON HIS FACE ⬭ This position
is not for everybody, but it is very erotic and
two people can have a lot of fun with it. The doer sits on
the man's face, facing his penis and genital area; her legs support her to
prevent excess weight from pressing on his head. From here the doer can
use hands and mouth to play with the doee's genitals. The doee's head
is supported by a pillow, and he can use his tongue and mouth on her
pussy and anus at the same time that she does him (FIGURE 4.10). This
can be a "coming together" posi-
tion, but in it the man
is unable to efficiently
use his hands.

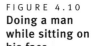

FIGURE 4.9
**Doing a man
while sitting
on your side**

FIGURE 4.10
**Doing a man
while sitting on
his face**

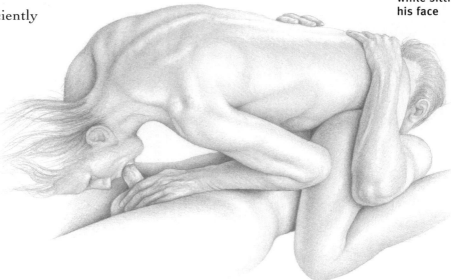

Coming Together

Before you attempt the positions described below, it is important that you are first able to give and receive pleasure using one of the previously described positions. You will more successfully learn EMO when both you and your partner put all of your attention on one orgasm at a time. Then, once you become adept at giving and receiving EMOs, you may wish to check out these "coming together" positions. The better you get at giving each other an orgasm one at a time, the easier it will be to come together.

Remember, too, that two people who want to come together can use any position they can invent that gives both partners access to each other's genitals.

"TWO-HEADED MONSTER" 🖎 This position (FIGURE 4.11), which is similar to the sixty-nine position, was named by Dr. Vic Baranco. The woman lies on her back on a comfortable surface. The man begins the action just as he would in the "lying on your side" position, described above. That is, he lies with his head in the opposite direction from hers. Make sure each person has enough pillows in all the necessary sizes to remain comfortable for an extended time, and be sure that sufficient lubricant is easily accessible to each person. The man may want pillows against his back to help him stay propped up. A pillow can be placed over the woman's thigh, as described in the "lying on your side" position. The man may want a pillow placed on the

FIGURE 4.11
"Two-headed monster" position

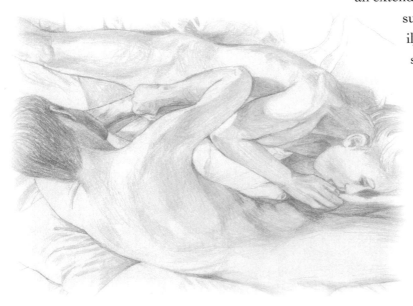

woman's abdomen on which to rest his forearm and elbow, especially if he is bony. He also may tuck a small pillow into his armpit for added comfort.

The man stimulates the woman until she is getting off well; then she rolls onto her side and takes the man's genitals in her hands. She may want to use a pillow so she can rest her torso on his thigh, as well as a couple of larger pillows placed at her back so she can remain easily propped up. Once both partners are feeling good, the man may wish to roll onto his back to relax still more. She might put the head of his penis in her mouth as she continues to rub with her hands.

Since both partners are lying on the same side, with the same hand free, this position works best if both have the same dominant hand (both are right-handed or both are left-handed). If one is left-handed and the other right-handed, they have to decide which person will use the weaker hand as the doing hand. In an additional maneuver (workable if your bed is large enough), the man can place the pillows supporting his back against the wall or headboard. This provides greater support for his back.

Besides the divided attention, the two-headed monster's biggest difficulty is getting both partners comfortable in the position. It works best if both people put all of their attention on either their own or their partner's genitals. The way to accomplish this is to make sure that all the other body parts—such as legs, arms, and back—are in a relaxed, stress-free state, requiring no extra attention. Take as much time as necessary to get the pillows and your bodies in the right position.

BONOBO POSITION We named this position after the bonobos, or pygmy chimps, who are very promiscuous, although we have never heard of a bonobo actually using this position. (They might if they saw two humans use it, but they would probably call it the "human position.") Start out as in the sitting position (described earlier), with the woman lying down; after a while the woman extends her arms and starts playing with the man's genitals as he continues to rub hers. She remains prone and he remains sitting up; he must therefore make sure that he can stay relaxed in this position. The man

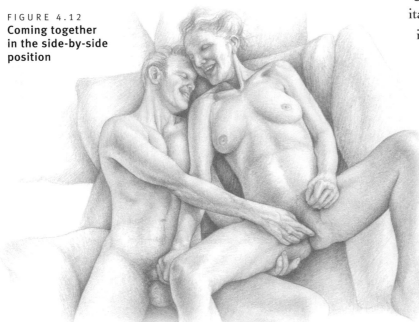

FIGURE 4.12
Coming together in the side-by-side position

has great visual access to her genitals, but the woman has a limited view of his. This works out okay, as she has no difficulty finding the penis.

SIDE BY SIDE ⬧ Refer to the descriptions of this position in the sections "Doing a Woman" and "Doing a Man," above. It can be modified to allow both partners to stimulate each other's genitals. With this position, neither partner has good visual access to the other's genitals, but because of the face-to-face contact, it is quite intimate (FIGURE 4.12).

⬧ Positioning the Hands ⬧

FOR DOING A WOMAN ⬧ First, we are going to describe how to do a woman's genitals—without actually involving the woman. Men feel so much mystery and confusion about women's genitals that it is easier initially to discuss them in the absence of any real-life examples. If you have never actually seen a woman's vulva, it would make sense to first learn about female anatomy from a book. If you have never touched a woman's genitals in good lighting with the goal of giving her an intense orgasm, it might help to practice some of the techniques described below on your own before actually confronting those mysterious body parts in person.

We use the eraser end of an unsharpened pencil as our model. This is a technique we use when we have a new student who wishes to learn the art of clitoral stimulation. (Once again, we would like to thank Dr. Vic Baranco for suggesting this idea.) This teaching tool has proven very effective in giving students confidence and an understanding of what they will be doing. It allows the student to learn how to correctly position his hand and fingers without having to worry about a live woman's response to his initial mistakes and adjustments. His fear, excitement, and confusion over her mysterious vulva do not get in the way of his learning the proper techniques. Once he has mastered the techniques—including anchoring the clitoris, retracting the hood, stroking the clitoris, and even making some verbal communications— on a pencil, the student is allowed to practice on a real woman and her real clitoris and vulva.

Although a woman who is learning to do another woman will not experience the mystery that a man confronts about a woman's genitals, she still must learn the proper techniques. She has to become skilled at the specific placement of her hands. Additionally, it is easier, at first, to practice one's communication skills on an inanimate object, as long as one is taking the exercise seriously. For these reasons, it is a good idea for even a woman who wishes to learn to rub other women to begin with a pencil.

As the doer, you get the most out of the experience when you touch to enjoy the feelings and the sensations in the hand (or any other body part) that you're using to touch. When you do this, you're living in the moment, as close to the present as possible. This is what sensuality is all about: feeling whatever is happening, in the most pleasurable way—even if it is with a pencil eraser.

Begin by enjoying the pencil as much as possible; observe its texture, its firmness, whatever. Learn to touch it and talk to it as if it were a beautiful woman. Your hand is a sex organ, touching only for pleasure. Practice talking to the pencil about what you feel, how beautiful she is, and any changes you can imagine noticing. Practice giving it acknowledgments and commands (see "Ideas for Communication," in the back of the book). Fantasize; make something up to rehearse your talking skills.

You can have fun with a pencil and eraser, or you can think this exercise is silly and superfluous. But the more fun you can have with a pencil, the more fun you will have when you get your hands on the real thing. No matter what, you eventually will have to practice on a real live woman; but the more confidence you can learn with a pencil, the more at ease and in control you will be when you rub a woman.

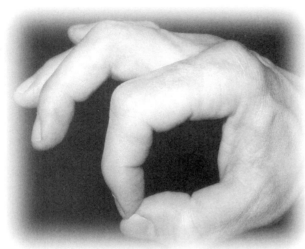

FIGURE 4.13
Position of right hand, demonstrating hooking of index finger and closeness of index finger to thumb

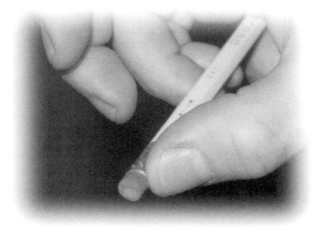

FIGURE 4.14
Placement of right thumb on eraser

Before you begin touching the pencil, look at FIGURE 4.13 to see how to hold your fingers for a right-handed "do."

If you are right-handed, hold the pencil in your left hand, with the eraser pointing downward and away from your body. Now take your right thumb and place it firmly along the left side of the pencil where metal meets eraser (FIGURE 4.14). Imagine that the eraser is the head of the clitoris. The metal part is equivalent to the pulled-back hood and the shaft of the clitoris. Pretend that the metal part was covering the eraser, and that the thumb has retracted this covering and now is anchoring the hood and the shaft of the clitoris.

Now that the eraser or clitoris is exposed, you can place the index or middle finger of your right hand on the upper left quadrant of the eraser (FIGURES 4.15, 4.16, AND 4.17).

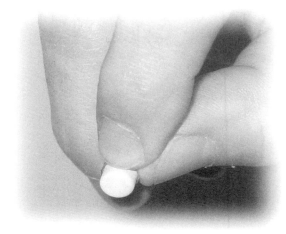

FIGURE 4.15
Right index finger stroking upper left quadrant of eraser. Notice proximity of thumb

We focus here on the upper left quadrant of the eraser because, on most women, the upper left quadrant of the clitoris is its most sensitive spot. Imagine that the clitoris is the face of a clock; if you looked at the clock straight on, most women's "hot spot" would be located at approximately 1:30. From the viewer's perspective, this is the upper right quadrant; from the woman's perspective, it's the upper left quadrant.

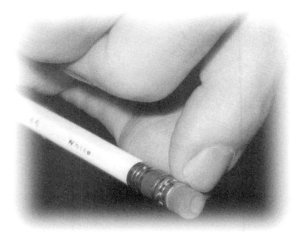

FIGURE 4.16
Another angle of right index finger stroking upper left quadrant of eraser

Begin stroking the eraser with a short up-and-down stroke. Use an almost pinching motion with your finger, as if you were picking up a piece of paper. In order to get the best angle on the upper left quadrant of the eraser/clitoris, you might need to tilt

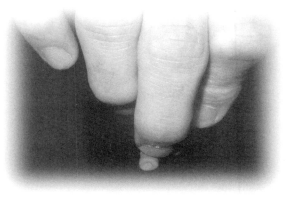

FIGURE 4.17
Right middle finger stroking upper left quadrant of eraser

your hand toward the left, as if you were reading your watch (FIGURE 4.18). You can rest your elbow on the edge of a desk or table if you will be practicing for an extended time.

If you are left-handed, hold the pencil in your right hand, again with the eraser pointing downward and away from you. Place the thumb of your left hand firmly along the right side of the pencil, where eraser and metal join (FIGURE 4.19). Pretend to retract the covering of the eraser/clitoris with your thumb and anchor the metal part/shaft of the clitoris at the same time. Now that the eraser/clitoris is exposed, you can use the index or middle finger of your left hand to begin stroking the upper left quadrant of the eraser (FIGURES 4.20 AND 4.21). Your hand should already be in the correct position; you won't have to tilt it as right-handed people do. The motion again is a pinching one; your thumb and finger are separated by the width of the eraser.

Once you have mastered this technique, you can take your pencil for peaks. Play with all different kinds of strokes, speeds, and pressures. Continue to practice talking to the pencil, and take breaks when it feels right. Retracting the hood, anchoring with the thumb, and the tilt of the

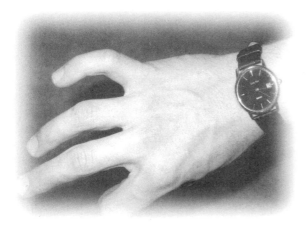

FIGURE 4.18
Tilting of hand and wrist of right hand to obtain proper angle to stroke left side of clitoris, like looking at your watch

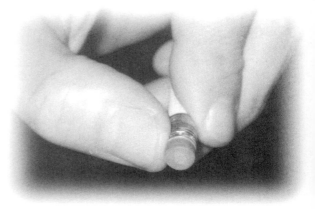

FIGURE 4.19
Placement of left thumb

hand (if you are right-handed) are some of the most difficult physical techniques to master in the art of doing. Getting practice here will make the
adjustment to real female genitals much easier. However, since the "hood"
of the eraser is already "pulled back" when you start, you will have to
learn how to pull back the hood when you are doing a real woman. As we
state in the "Genital Anatomy" chapter, every woman's hood is unique; the
retractability of each varies. This is such an important issue that we devote
a whole section to it (see the "Clitoral Hood" section of that chapter).

Once the student has the knack of how to hold his or her hand, we
often graduate them to a real woman's body. Sometimes this requires only
a few minutes. We graduate them quickly because they are paying a large
sum of money to take the course and need to progress; it does not mean
they should never use the pencil again. We encourage students to take
their pencils home and continue to practice on them. Doing so allows them
to continue to learn better communication skills and to become more
relaxed and proficient at correctly positioning their hands. A person who
is reading this book can take more time with the pencil before practicing
on a woman. It is best if your hands can really become comfortable in this

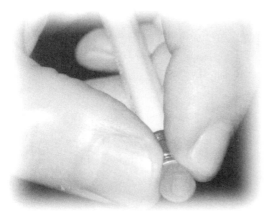

FIGURE 4.20
**Placement of
left index finger
on upper left
side of eraser**

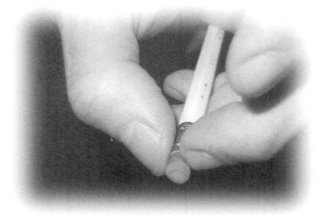

FIGURE 4.21
**Placement of left
middle finger on
upper left quad-
rant of eraser**

new position so that when you do touch a woman you will not feel awkward. And the more you can practice talking while doing a pencil, the better you will be at talking when it counts.

FOR DOING A MAN   Once you learn how to touch and stroke a penis, you'll discover how much fun you can have with it. Above we recommended that readers learning to do women first practice on a pencil eraser. Practicing is helpful, too, for those learning to do men. Select an object of similar shape, such as a dildo, a cucumber, or a banana. It is best to approach a penis with confidence and, of course, to touch it for your own pleasure, so think about these things when practicing on the object. A good first exercise is found in Chapter 2: try different ways of lubricating the object. Practice your communication skills, too. You might feel a little silly, but these objects are less charged than an actual penis and, by using them, you can practice your communication skills and learn how to touch in a way that makes your hand feel wonderful. Take ownership of the object—and, later, the penis—as if it belonged to you and you know just how to please it. A penis can respond with pleasure to almost any kind of touch that is done sensually.

After you're comfortable with your object practice, you can try your skills on a real person. As in doing a woman, when doing a man, remember that it is important to touch for your own pleasure. Hold your hand in a comfortable position, one that will allow you to stroke continuously for a number of minutes.

Before taking hold of the penis, make friends with it. Look at it. Notice if there are any loose pubic hairs, and remove them. Gently brush aside any attached pubic hairs, so that what you will be stroking is smooth. Hairs may fall off and attach themselves to your hand or his penis while you stroke. Any time you notice a loose hair, communicate and remove it quickly. An irritating pubic hair can mean the difference between your partner's great orgasm and his never wanting you to touch him again.

Once you're ready to start stroking, there are many different strokes you can try: turn to the "Giving an EMO" chapter to read about them. We usually recommend, when starting, that you use your full hand, with as much of the hand's surface in contact with the penis as possible. Circle the base of the penis with your second (nondoing) hand to hold the penis steady, and then grasp the penis with your whole doing hand. Position the doing hand with its thumb pointed upward, with as much of your fingertips as possible in contact with the urethra that is running along the center of the underside—from the base to the head—of his penis (see FIGURE 4.22). If the man is uncircumcised (as we mention in the "Genital Anatomy" chapter), you can also pull down his foreskin with this grasp. Stroke in an up-and-down movement, feeling your hand move against his penis in both directions.

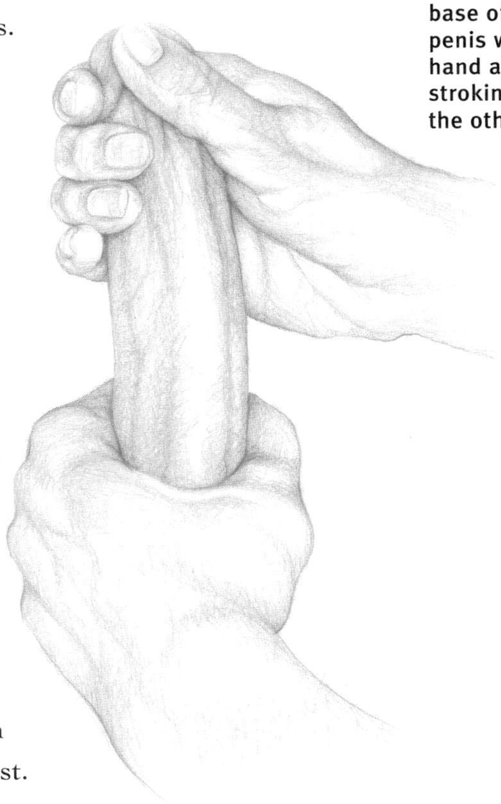

FIGURE 4.22
Holding the base of the penis with one hand and stroking with the other

Different men prefer different pressures. When you first take hold of the penis, do so with a sure touch. The pressure to use thereafter varies depending on what you have learned from touching him before. If you are unsure, or if you have never touched this man before, it is best to start with a fairly firm, medium-pressure stroke. You do not want to start too lightly, as you might seem tentative. You do not want to start with too much pressure, as you do not want to scare him. It's like "Goldilocks and the Three Bears"; you want to touch him just right. The right pressure is similar to a good handshake; you do not want to squeeze the other person's hand too much, nor do you want to be too wimpy. Once you get him going, you can use whatever pressure feels best.

Now that we have provided you with information on how to tease your partner, and on genital anatomy and body and hand positioning, we are almost ready to describe doing in detail. However, before we jump to the chapters that describe how to actually give and receive orgasms, we want you to become intimately familiar with your own body and learn what feels best to you. Accordingly, the next chapter is about masturbation, and it includes numerous exercises that will provide you with the self-knowledge you need to tell your partner, in detail, about what turns you on—and to present your partner with the gift of your turned-on body.

CHAPTER FIVE

Masturbation and Guilt   Masturbation has been given a bad rap. The word itself is derived from Latin and means "to defile or dishonor by hand." People have been led to believe that if they masturbate, they will go blind or grow hair on their palms, so that everyone will see what "dirty business" they'd been up to. Many religions consider "self abuse" sinful and to be avoided. Yet almost everyone masturbates anyway.

Masturbation

Unfortunately, when many people masturbate, they fail to take the most possible pleasure from the act. They do it, believe they are wrong for doing it, and feel guilty afterward. They do it to relieve themselves of the pressure of their tumescence, without taking the time to feel each stroke. Masturbation is a goal-oriented activity for many, and as a result the pleasure derived from it is minimal.

The reasons that different cultures and societies have frowned upon masturbation—and all other pleasurable pursuits—are quite complex. Millennia ago, when humans lived in small tribes as hunter-gatherers and were threatened regularly by other tribes and wild animals, survival was the highest priority, and so people could not hold the pursuit of pleasure—including masturbation—as a high priority. We live in a different world now, one where we hope pleasure will take a higher priority.

Women have come in for some of the worst of worldwide prejudice against sexual pleasure. Women had their clitorises removed, in a procedure called *clitoridectomy,* as late as the turn of the last century in this country; the patriarchal societies of some African and Middle Eastern countries still engage in this cruel practice. In medieval Europe, some women had to wear chastity belts. As a result of such customs, women, even more than men, had to squelch their sexual desires and thoughts.

According to Nancy Friday, in her book *Women on Top,* the American Medical Association pronounced masturbation "normal" only in 1972. Women in the 1950s and early '60s generally did not even admit to having sexual fantasies, let alone to masturbating. Women were regarded as either the Madonna or the prostitute; most were considered to be practically asexual.

Masturbation, in American society, has also been frowned upon because of the inherent link between it and fantasy: masturbation usually accompanies sexual fantasy. According to Friday, the "sin" of sexual thoughts and fantasies was considered even greater than the "sin" of actual masturbatory hand on the genitals. The hand's motion was just a mechanical act, but the thoughts were part of the person's identity. People's guilt about masturbation was reinforced by the conditioning of parents and religious leaders, which (although fantasies are purely mental and cannot be physically taken away) tended to stifle the imagination. In the past, women who did admit to having fantasies often talked about the "rape" fantasy. Imagining that sex was done to them without their consent was the easiest way that they could handle their guilt about their sexual thoughts. This did not mean these women actually wished to be raped, only that such a fantasy felt safest to their psyches. Especially in our society, this anti-pleasure and anti-masturbation attitude has been slowly changing in the last few decades, thanks to pioneering teachers of sensuality such as Betty Dodson, Dr. Vic Baranco, Earle Milliard Marsh, M.D., and, of course, Masters and Johnson. According to Friday, women of the 1980s and '90s indulged in a much wider range of sexual fantasies, and women became more willing to admit to them. Women nowadays admit to having fantasies about other women and about being in sexual control of men—hence the title of her book *Women on Top*.

Children, as well as adult men and women, sometimes masturbate. We believe it is quite normal for some children to enjoy touching themselves for pleasure. In the past, and occasionally in this day and age, some children have been yelled at or even spanked for touching themselves on their own genitals. This is simply an example of parents repeating the way that they were treated when they were children (and it is in keeping with the whole negative stereotype about masturbation). At the beginning of the twenty-first century, we hope people are becoming more enlightened on this topic. But because our society is so conditioned against children's recognition of their sexuality, it is best to let kids know that if they are going to touch themselves, they should do it in a private place, such as the bathroom. It is also all right if children do *not* masturbate or touch themselves. After puberty, they'll have plenty of time to learn more about this option. At the other extreme, some parents in other cultures rub their children's genitals to keep the kids calm and happy. This is probably not too common, but it reveals that human behavior and rules can vary widely, depending on location and culture.

Learning to Masturbate

We believe that masturbation is not only one of the most enjoyable ways to be pleasured but also is a necessary part of learning the intricacies of your nervous system and how it can be stimulated for optimum pleasure. Once you know how best to be pleasured, you can relate the information to your partner, so he or she can take you to the next level of pleasure.

In this chapter, we explore the fun of masturbating both by yourself and with your partner. We present a series of exercises designed to help you actually become better at masturbating. The exercises are best done on your own at first, so that all your attention is focused on yourself and your own pleasure. Later, you may be able to incorporate some of these exercises into your love life with another.

To become good at almost anything, you have to practice. To gain knowledge in a certain area, you have to do research. The following exercises, more than any other techniques we teach, have helped numerous students of sensuality to learn more about, and to love, their bodies. The exercises have changed many a person's life for the better, starting the very first time they did them. We have graduate students — some of whom have gone on to teach sensuality themselves — who regularly practice these very same exercises.

We included these exercises in our first book. However, we are taking advantage of this opportunity to write afresh about them. The exercises are such that they can always teach you something new about yourself; all you need is interest, curiosity, and creativity.

A word of advice: Do the exercises in the order presented here. The exercise that deals directly with masturbation is preceded by four important exercises that, if done in proper order, will enhance your masturbatory sensations.

Visiting Dignitary

The goal of this exercise is to learn to treat yourself better than you usually do. We've given it this name because most people, if told that a special dignitary was coming for a visit, would make an extra effort to prepare for and entertain that dignitary. Most of us—especially men, but plenty of women, too—pay little attention to creating a pleasurably sensual environment. And even if you already hold a high opinion of yourself and treat yourself accordingly, there is always something extra you can do to create a little more pleasure for yourself.

Imagine that a famous person—someone you admire—is coming to visit you. This can be your favorite movie star, a politician, or a member of the British royal family. First, pick a place where you'll entertain your special guest. This is usually the bedroom, but we have known students who have put a soft rug before the living-room fireplace or even turned their bathroom into a pleasure zone. Now get the chosen area ready for your visiting dignitary. Clean up the space so it looks appreciably better. You don't have to sand the floors or polish the furniture or spend hours at the task; just make it as nice as possible in a reasonable amount of time.

As it turns out, the visiting dignitary is *you*. You are the special person on whom this attention is to be showered. While cleaning your chosen room or even beforehand, think of what you would like to use for pleasuring each one of your senses. Some or all of these items might be in your house already, or you may want to go out for a little shopping trip. Make sure your room is properly heated. We have known students who tried these exercises in rooms that were too cold; of course, they failed to enjoy themselves as much as they could have.

Choose an item whose fragrance you really enjoy. You can use scented oils, incense, a scented candle, a fragrant flower, perfume, your lover's panties, or whatever you like. According to David Sobel and Robert Ornstein in *Healthy Pleasures,* the sense of smell is our most ignored and underappreciated sense. Smell is connected to the emotion-generating areas of our brain; both are located in the limbic system. Smell, therefore, can have a great subconscious influence on our moods, behaviors, and memories. Sexual desire and the "fight or flight" response are also located close to the rhinencephalon (nose-brain) in the limbic system. It is no wonder that smells have such a powerful influence on how we feel.

Select some of your favorite foods. Bear in mind that you do not want to consume a big meal before or during your sensual practice. You might make a fruit plate with your favorite seasonal delicacies, or choose a few pieces of chocolate—dark, light, or truffles. You could select nuts, cheeses, ice cream—whatever you fancy. Vera likes to use dark chocolate and berries.

Get something to drink. It could be your favorite juice, or a carbonated beverage. One glass of wine or champagne is the maximum, as alcohol desensitizes the nerve endings. Some people choose their favorite bottled water. It is also a good idea to use a flexible straw to make drinking easier, especially since your hands will be full of lubricant.

Now make sure that you have something you enjoy looking at. It could be a bouquet of flowers, a pretty candle, a beautiful painting, or a fireplace. Again, the choice is yours, and you can choose different objects each time you do these exercises. You can also use the same object for more than one sense.

To please your sense of hearing, listen to your favorite music. Some people make special tapes or program their CD players to play certain pieces. We had a student who used the classical piece "Bolero" to peak himself over and over again. Other people have used sounds of birds outside their window, a running brook, or ocean waves splashing on a beach.

Find something that feels great to touch. It could be an item of silk, satin, or velvet clothing. It could be a smooth sculpture, a feather, or whatever.

For your final sense, which is your conceptual thought, you can introduce any idea, concept, or entertainment that stimulates your eroticism. You can play a sexy video or read a romance novel or an erotic magazine. You can even use your own fantasy as a stimulant.

This exercise prepares you for the remaining exercises below. Once you have created your ideal sensual space for you, the "visiting dignitary," you are ready to continue with the remaining exercises. First, make sure you have a few necessary items: you will need a full-length mirror, a hand mirror, and your favorite lubricant. (Vaseline is excellent for masturbating. For other ideas, check out the "Lubricants" section in the "Teasing" chapter.) For the

"Tactile Inventory" exercise, the "Focal Point" exercise, "Connections," and masturbation itself, you usually will be lying down, so put your drink on a tray, table, or shelf close to where you'll lie down—if you get thirsty, you will not have to get up. (You'll be standing up for the first exercise, "Visual Inventory.") It is also best to set your CD player for continuous play so that you will not have to get up to change it. Make sure that you will not be disturbed for the duration of your special experience. Turn off the ringer on the phone, and put a sign on your door if you live with someone. Tell anyone who might enter your space that you wish not to be disturbed for the next hour or two.

Visual Inventory

Now that you have your space prepared, it is time to take advantage of it. The goal of this exercise is to learn to like and even love the way you look. The way to reach this goal is to look at yourself with admiring eyes. Usually, when we look at ourselves in the mirror, we look for what is wrong. We check for zits or bad hair; women might study their reflections for flaws in their makeup. In this exercise, you are to look at yourself only with admiration and appreciation. Look at yourself directly, using both the full-length mirror and the handheld mirror.

We usually recommend doing this exercise in full light, but you can use candlelight if you find it more flattering. Start by looking in the mirror at one part of yourself that you like, and put your total visual attention there. You will find that you like likeable things even more when you focus attention on them. Then move your attention to another area and appreciate it. Once you identify one area that you like, you will find it easier to locate another one. Some students like to do a little striptease for themselves, taking off one piece of clothing at a time. Take your time. and move from one part of your body to another. Look at the shape, color, and musculature—anything you like.

Do not spend any time looking at an area if you don't like it, but remember that it is possible to change your mind about your body when you see it through admiring eyes. We knew someone who had a scar he'd always hated; doing this exercise, he found it beautiful and unique. This person learned to love what previously he could not stand. Another student, who disliked his fat belly, learned to appreciate it. The more you get into the habit of viewing yourself with positive eyes, the easier it becomes. Not only will you find yourself more attractive, but other people will notice a positive change in you too. You will be more turned on and have more sex appeal.

Use both mirrors at once to check out areas that you don't usually see, such as the backs of your knees and arms, and your anus. Check out your genitals with and without a mirror. Notice the different colors of your skin there, any movement of your body, or changes you might not have noticed. We have come across more than one student who had never really looked at their genitals. Later on, after you have been masturbating for a while, you can check out your genitals again with the hand mirror and notice any changes that have occurred, so keep your mirror handy.

Take as much time with this exercise as you like. It's best to do what feels best. You can take breaks at any time to taste, smell, listen, or indulge whatever senses you would like to stimulate. Then go back to the mirror with new energy and vigor. Create any kind of visual stimulus you can think of to add to your enjoyment of yourself, including viewing yourself from many different angles and positions.

This is a great exercise to use in combination with the other ones given here, and it also can be used and enjoyed on its own. You can do it before taking a bath or a shower. Learn to love your body, with all its marks and scars, and not only will you exude more sex appeal, but you will actually become more and more beautiful.

Tactile Inventory

The goal of this exercise is to learn how and where you prefer to be touched. We originally called it "pinch and scratch" because it calls for touching yourself all over your body with all kinds of touches. Anything is acceptable —

light touches, firm touches, pinching, scratching with the nails, stroking with the back of the hand, and any other way of touching yourself that you can imagine. The only rule is that the touch be pleasurable. You can go as light or as heavy as you wish to test the limits of your pleasure. You'll find that different parts of your body like different types of pressure. You might prefer a light stroke on your nipple and a firmer one on your shoulder. The inside, protected areas usually are more sensitive than outer ones — for example, you can squeeze your outer elbow with much more pressure than your inner elbow will enjoy.

Again, do this exercise for as long as it is fun and you enjoy it. There is no set amount of time that you must spend on it. You can take breaks whenever you desire; then try checking out a new and different touch after your break.

Focal-Point Exercise

This is really part of your tactile inventory. The goal of this exercise is to deliberately tumesce, or sensually arouse, a selected area of your body. First, choose a sensitive spot on your body, such as a nipple, the inner elbow, a spot on your lip, or wherever. Then, with your hand, lightly stroke the area surrounding the selected spot. We recommend using concentric circles that approach and then move away from the spot over and over again, without touching the spot itself. A fairly quick and light stroke usually works best when you wish to increase the tumescence. As the tumescence builds, you will have the urge to touch the avoided spot. Continue teasing yourself as long as your sensation remains on this side of torture. When you cannot take it any longer, firmly rub the whole area, slowly, including the spot, to detumesce the area.

You can do this exercise on more than one spot. You can try out different lubricants to see how you like them. You can do one nipple with lubricant and the other without lubricant and compare the two sensations. Do as much or as little as you prefer, taking as many breaks as you like.

⟡ Masturbation Itself ⟡

When we assign this exercise in our class, we call it "masturbation for pleasurable effect." We tell the students they are not allowed to climax ("squirt" or go over the edge) while they are doing their homework. The reason: Most people masturbate to relieve tension, not necessarily to extend their pleasure over time. And most people feel pressure to have an orgasm/ejaculation as "proof" that they've succeeded, and we do not want to add to this pressure. The goal of this exercise is to have as much fun and pleasure as possible, and to extend this pleasure as long as possible through the use of peaking.

For our men readers: whether you squirt at the end is entirely up to you, but it is not part of the goal when you are starting out. As you get more relaxed and proficient at going for the pleasure instead of the squirt, we would like for you to play with the ejaculatory phase and to become skilled at getting close to the edge and even going for the big ejaculation.

In the following paragraphs, we describe and illustrate masturbation techniques that have worked for us and for our students. When you do the above exercises before masturbating, you are creating an atmosphere that makes you conducive to receiving the most pleasure from your body. By treating yourself royally, with a nice space and lots of pleasurable stimulants around you, you treat yourself better than usual; this allows you to feel more. By doing the visual inventory, you learn to love yourself more, becoming more turned on to yourself and gaining new sex appeal. The combination of the visual and tactile inventories is meant to tumesce you into a higher state of pleasure. Then, when you begin to masturbate, you are primed for a great time. People are often victimized by time; they never seem to have enough time to do the things that they think they want to do. If this is the case, it is okay to masturbate without doing all of the above exercises or after doing only some of them. We highly recommend that you do the entire series of exercises, in order, at least some of the time, if not every time.

Even if you don't have much available time, still take the time to set up your space with a few extra touches, such as something tasty to drink or eat and some nice music. This takes only a few seconds; from there, you can go right into touching your erogenous areas.

FOR WOMEN ✍ Get into a comfortable position, such as lying on your back on a bed. Use as many pillows as necessary to make yourself comfortable, so that you are relaxed all over and most of your energy can be used for feeling and touching your genitals. Make sure your drink, lubricant, and towels are nearby.

If you have done all the exercises described above, you are probably tingling by now. Take your time, depending on how much time you have available, and lightly play with your pubic hair and vulva area. Get it feeling so good down there that your clitoris is itching to be touched. You cannot tease yourself as well as someone else can, but you still can have a lot of fun playing. Choose your clitoris as the focal point; touch everything around it except the clitoris itself. Sometimes you may want to forego the teasing and go straight for your spot to get the orgasm on a fast track. Again, the choice to do this depends on how much time you wish to spend and how tumesced you feel. If you're taking it slowly, lubricate as much of your vulva area as you wish, excluding the clitoris, which you are still teasing and holding out on. If you are taking the fast track, then make sure your clitoris is lubricated, too.

Touch yourself—on the clitoris or elsewhere—to feel the most pleasure you can at that moment. Once you've reached your favorite spot on the clitoris, usually by pulling back on the hood with your palm (see the explanation of how to do this in the "Genital Anatomy" chapter), it is best to choose one continuous type of stroke, using your index or middle finger on your favorite spot (FIGURE 5.1). For most women, as we said earlier in the book, that favorite spot is the upper left quadrant of the clitoris. We recommend a short up-and-down stroke.

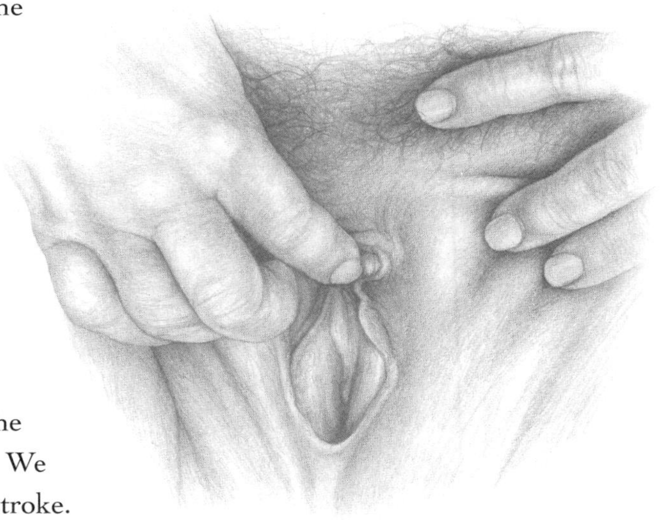

FIGURE 5.1
Woman masturbating with index finger on her clitoris

If you have another favorite area, it is fine to touch and peak yourself there, but we would like you to at least check out the upper left quadrant of your clitoris at some point during this exercise.

Some women may be used to masturbating with a different type of stroke or with a vibrator. This new up-and-down stroke on the left side may not, at least at first, feel as good as your old way of doing it. The goal of this masturbation exercise is pleasure, and although we do want it to feel as good as possible to you, we're also asking you to explore and possibly to find a new and better way to do it. Vibrators, although efficient in the production of an orgasm, tend to numb your clitoris to the touch of your own or someone else's hand and to any kind of stimulus except a vibrator. Therefore, unless you are married to your vibrator and do not want to have other lovers or to experience the most pleasure from your own hand, we think you're best served by moving away from your reliance on it.

In addition to doing the stroke described above, feel free to touch any part of your vulva or clitoris that feels good to you. If you never have masturbated or are used to a vibrator, your clitoris and entire vulva area may not feel much sensation at first. There are a lot of nerve endings in this area, however, so if you put your attention on the stroke, you will be able to feel something. It may not be as much or as intense as you had hoped for, but approve of any sensation that you do feel. Keep doing the same stroke over and over, as long as it feels good.

When you have had enough of one stroke, take a break or start doing another stroke. The moment that you sense that the next stroke will be even slightly less exquisite than the last, you have peaked, or reached the highest point in that orgasmic cycle. At this point, experiment with deliberately taking the orgasm down a notch or two; you do this by changing the stroke.

You do not have to keep stroking the upper left quadrant for every peak. Feel free to do whatever you can think of that feels good. Check out different parts of your clitoris. Check out touching yourself with different speeds and different pressures. This is your time to research the entire gamut of possible sensations. Find out what you like best. Refer to the "Giving an EMO" chapter, later in this book, where we describe a variety of strokes, many of which you can do on yourself. Once your clitoris is engorged and retracted from its hood, your other hand is free to explore areas inside and outside your vagina. (Read the "Insertion" chapter to learn more about the interior of the vagina or anus.) You can play with your labia and perineum while simultaneously stroking your clitoris. Play with yourself as long as you like. You are not rubbing to set time records, but for the fun of it and to learn how you like to be touched. Peak yourself often, and see if you can take yourself higher than before.

As you do this exercise, it's likely that you may feel more—or at least differently—than you did when you masturbated in the usual, "tensed-up" state. Remember that you're learning about a different kind of orgasm: an EMO. Notice and approve of every stroke, and see if you can feel any contractions or other signs of orgasm. Check to see if you can feel that first stroke and be in orgasm from the start of the exercise. Remember that the immediate goal is to feel pleasure, not to put yourself under stress or to imagine that you have to feel "a certain amount" or else feel like you've lost. The ultimate goal may be to have a long and intense orgasm, but the best way to get there is with small, approving steps.

WATER MASSAGE There is another way a woman can masturbate that allows her to feel as if she is being done to, rather than feeling that she's doing it to herself. This may seem similar to the use of a vibrator, but it does not numb the nerve endings as a vibrator does. This method calls for allowing water to massage the genitals, specifically the clitoris. If you have access to a bidet, you can sit on it, adjust the water pressure and temperature, and position your vulva so that the water hits your clitoris in a pleasurable and titillating way. Some Jacuzzis and swimming pools have water jets against which you can position your vulva to allow the stream of water to pleasurably massage you. (You probably do not want to do this when other people are around!) Many of the jets are either too strong or at a bad angle, but occasionally you may find one that works for you.

A more reliable and private way to enjoy a water massage on your genitals is to equip your bathtub with a hose. Some faucets permit you to fasten a simple hand-shower attachment; just cut off the large shower end so that the open hose is attached to the faucet. However, these hand-shower attachments do not fit many modern bathroom fixtures. In that case, you can go to Home Depot or someplace similar to get the appropriate hose and hardware; with some minor plumbing skills, these can be attached to the rear of your regular shower head.

Once you have your hose in place, fill your tub with enough warm water to lie in, but not enough to cover your genitals. You can bring in as much of the "visiting dignitary" stuff as you like, such as music and something to drink. Now lie back in the tub and point the water from the hose at your vulva. Aim it at your clitoris or wherever you like. Adjust the water pressure and temperature to suit your preference. You can squeeze the end of the hose if you want to get a finer and higher-pressured stream. Play with the water; peak yourself as often as you like.

Many of our students really enjoy this water-massage technique and use it regularly. Some people like to get themselves off with this method before they do their partner; that way, they don't feel needy and can focus all their attention on the other person.

FOR MEN ❧ You have done the first four exercises and you are turned on and ready. You have treated yourself royally and enjoyed the process. Get in a comfortable position; lie down with pillows placed in the proper positions to support your body for an extended period. Pillows placed under the legs, head, and neck are usually helpful, although individual preferences vary. Make sure that your necessary accessories are close by. These include lubricant, towels, and a drink.

Begin by lightly tickling your body; work your way toward the genital area. Lightly play with your pubic hair, and move your hands around your genitals with light strokes. Your penis may or may not be hard; in either case, you can now take your favorite lubricant and gently lubricate your penis. I like using Vaseline, as I need to apply it only once. I like to put it on the back and bottom of my penis first, and work it around to the underside and finally to the apex and head of my cock. (The "bottom" of the penis is actually the part of the shaft closest to the body. The "back" of the penis is the side that's visible when the penis is flaccid. The "underside" is the side that lies against the scrotum when the penis is flaccid and that, in erection, becomes the visible side.) Sometimes I like to put it on slowly, other times quickly. You can apply it with one finger or with your whole hand. Make sure all the parts of your penis are coated with lubricant.

Masturbation can be a time of exploration and learning. Check out all kinds of strokes and touches. Wrap the palm of your hand around your penis, making as much contact as possible between your hand and penis. Squeeze to see what kinds of pressure feel good. The harder and more turned on you are, the more pressure you can usually take, although more pressure may not necessarily afford the most pleasure. Try squeezing and releasing, then repeat this pattern. Try long strokes from the base of the penis to the tip, feeling the pleasure and the stroke in both directions. Try repeating the same kind of stroke but use different speeds and pressures.

To bring yourself up, it is best to use a steady, repetitive stroke, so make sure you find one that feels really good. You can stroke just one finger up and down the underside of your penis (that is, the side that lies against the body when the penis is flaccid). You can use a short stroke just on the apex. You can do anything you like that feels good. This is your time to experiment and be creative. Check out as many types of touches and strokes as you can invent and enjoy.

The goal is to make each stroke feel as good as possible while building your tumescence as high as you can and remaining as relaxed as you can. Learning how high you can go without going over the edge requires experimenting with your body. Usually, before ejaculation, the penis goes into what is called a *secondary erection* (FIGURE 5.2). The head of the penis

FIGURE 5.2
Secondary erection

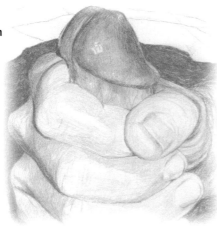

gets even larger, bulging out and turning deep purple. With enough practice, men can recognize when they are approaching this point of no return.

To become a master masturbator, you want to bring yourself as close to the edge as possible and then peak. To peak yourself, you have to change the stroke or stop stroking. This enables you to come down a bit so that you can start the next peak. Sometimes you might go on a little too long; if that happens, you can stop yourself from going over by either squeezing the head of the penis or pressing inward and upward in the area under the testicles, where the prostate and ejaculatory duct are located (FIGURE 5.3). You may actually see some ejaculate ooze out anyway, but not in an intense squirt. It is possible to experience orgasm, with contractions, seminal leakage, and intense pleasure, throughout this experience.

FIGURE 5.3
Pressing in under the scrotum

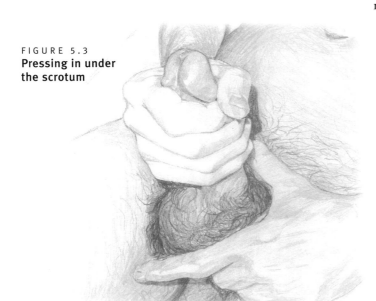

If you like, you can take breaks throughout this process. Once you've taken a break or peaked yourself, switch to another sort of steady stroke. You can add to the sensations by using your second hand to play with your testicles and with the part of your penis that is inside your body (what we call the "hidden cock"—see a fuller explanation in the "Genital Anatomy" chapter, earlier in the book). Pulling on the scrotal sack feels good, as does softly stroking it. Stroking the hidden cock at the same time that you stroke the penis can feel great. Your hand on the hidden-cock area is in a good position, too, to apply pressure to keep your-

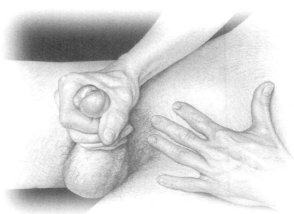

FIGURE 5.4
Adding pressure to abdominal area with second hand

self from going over. When you are high on a peak, placing your second hand on your lower abdominal area and exerting some pressure can add to your pleasure (FIGURE 5.4). Experiment with your second hand to see which strokes and touches feel best. Also check out the "Connections" exercise, below, to get more ideas for using your second hand.

To increase your pleasure while you are masturbating, you can use any form of conceptual thought or fantasy you like, including porno-graphic videos or maga-zines or simply mental fantasies. On the other hand, fantasizing is not required; feel free to choose whatever serves you best.

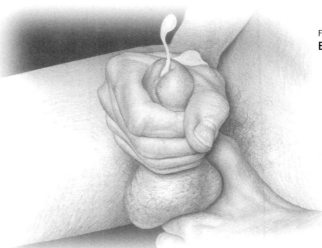

FIGURE 5.5
Ejaculation

A man can also experiment to see how he can feel the most pleasure during the actual ejaculatory phase (illustrated in FIGURE 5.5). He can play with pressure and speed to see what feels best as he continues to ejaculate. (We have found that progressively slowing and lightening the stroke usually feels best.) He can check out the "push out" technique right at the moment of ejaculation (see details on this tactic in the next chapter) to help extend his experience. Each person is different, so find out what works best for you. Do not worry if you mess up an ejaculation—we learn from our failures, and the next time you will do something different that will feel better.

Connections

The dermis, or skin, covers the entire body. Many touch receptors are located either in or close to the skin. The sense of touch is the first sense that has been reported to function in the developing fetus. When we are born, we can feel sensation all over our bodies. Many of these nerve receptors are connected, so a baby that's being tickled may feel the sensation all over its body. As we grow up, we learn to differentiate these sensations; we begin to associate different sensations with different body parts, and we learn to compartmentalize our body into specific parts.

Many of these nerves are still connected to one another, but most of us have not used these connections in years. Orgasm, for most people, is limited to a distinct sensation in the loins. However, it is possible to experience a total-body orgasm, or at least to feel the orgasm throughout parts of your body besides the genitals. The best way to spread the wonderful sensation of orgasm is by reconnecting or reawakening those connections. What follows is an exercise to help you do just that.

You can do this exercise after you finish masturbating or in the middle of masturbating. However, it is best not to have squirted or gone over the edge before doing the exercise, as at that point most people no longer want to continue touching themselves. Choose your favorite, most turned-on body part. This is usually the clitoris for women and the apex of the penis for men. We call this area the "primary area." Using lubricant, start stroking the primary area. Get it feeling really wonderful. Then choose a secondary area that you would like to connect to the primary area. Erectile tissues, such as a nipple, a lip, a labia, or the anus, are all quite sensitive and are good choices for your first connection.

Using lubricant, start stroking the secondary area as you continue to stroke the primary one. Stroke them in exactly the same way or as close to the same way as possible; that is, use the same speed, the same pressure, and the same length and direction of stroke. After getting both areas feeling great, lift your finger off the secondary area and continue to rub the primary one. Leave your finger hovering over the secondary area; you can even continue to do the same stroke in the air, without touching the skin.

Notice any sensation you feel in this secondary area. At first you might not feel very much. Some people report a slight sensation or a feeling of heat. As soon as the sensation goes away, put your finger back on the secondary area and again start stroking the two in sync.

Do this for a while, and then take your finger off the primary area. Again, you can keep stroking in the air above the primary area; just don't touch it. Notice any sensation you feel. When the sensation, if there is any, dies down, put your finger back on the primary area and continue stroking in sync. Keep doing this over and over again, on and off the secondary area, on and off the primary area. The longer you do this and the more often you do it, the stronger and more real the connection becomes. You can choose nonerectile tissue, too, as your secondary area—anything that feels good, such as an inner thigh, your belly, or even an earlobe.

Once you get a good connection going, it works in both directions. By connecting the lips of your mouth with your penis or your clitoris, you become that much more sensitive and feel that much more when you engage in kissing. You become able to stimulate your clitoris by touching your inner labia or introitus; this can greatly add to your enjoyment of intercourse, as you can feel sensation in your clitoris without being touched there. When you have an orgasm, you are able to feel it, to some extent, in your connected areas.

Although connecting different areas causes you to feel more, it is not, as some people would like to believe, a real substitute for directly stimulating the clitoris or the penis. To experience the best and most intense sensations, you still must directly engage those areas.

Becoming familiar with the various ways our bodies feel and look is vitally important to the serious student of sensuality. Besides helping you love yourself more, the basic tool of intimate knowledge of your body also equips you to be a better lover to someone else. The exercises in this chapter, created to increase your body awareness, bestow great benefits when they're done thoroughly and in the order they are presented. As we mentioned, however, you need not do all of them every time. It is okay, sometimes, to masturbate without first doing the inventories. But you get the most out of the exercises if you complete them in their entirety.

And, even though the exercises are designed to be done alone and without interruption, it might prove fun and informative to masturbate in front of your partner. By doing so, you can demonstrate to them some of the ways you have learned to pleasurably touch yourself—ways they can adopt later, when it is their turn to do you. It is always beneficial to show your partner how you peak yourself—and for men, specifically, to show their partners how to take them through an ejaculation (check out the final section of the next chapter, "Receiving an EMO," for more details about this skill). Likewise, you can also encourage your partner to masturbate in front of you, so you can learn from him or her. Some people may have strong conditioning against masturbating in front of someone, or against watching someone masturbate. If your partner expresses reservations, handle them gently and with love. Don't pressure your partner into doing it. Overcome these resistances by enjoying, playing with, and seducing your partner.

Now that we have researched our own bodies, we are in a great place to teach our partners how we like to be touched. The next chapter does just that.

CHAPTER SIX

In this chapter, we explore the best way to receive an orgasm. We present some hints to help you relax, and we discuss the importance of surrender. We describe the most effective communication techniques for getting your partner to touch you just right, with a special emphasis on the skills of acknowledgment and approval. We investigate the use of sexual fantasy as a technique to increase your pleasure. We deliberately did not separate this chapter into men's and women's sections because the best state for receiving an orgasm is the same for both sexes: relaxed and surrendered. Where applicable, we have addressed whatever gender-based specifics may exist.

Receiving an EMO

To experience an EMO, one of the most important things a person needs is the belief—or even better, the knowledge—that an EMO is possible. For that reason, it is quite valuable to witness a live demonstration of one, or at least a video. We hope the illustrations in this book will help prepare your mind for not only the possibility, but also the desirability, of an EMO.

Besides a belief in the possibility of an EMO, a desire to experience intense pleasure is also necessary. Once you become aware of the existence of EMOs, you still must aspire to actually having one. This can be accomplished by enthusiastically anticipating it. Whether your pleasure comes from your own hand or from the attention your partner focuses on you, your desire and pleasure manifest themselves if you willingly anticipate each stroke with as much of your consciousness as you can. It is also essential that you genuinely appreciate the amount of sensation you feel, no matter how small it may seem. This does not mean that you cannot aspire to feel more, but you need to get in agreement with the fact that you feel as much as you can at any given moment. Otherwise, if you're busy comparing levels of sensation from moment to moment, your mind is far away from the next stroke. Comparisons are beneficial to happiness only if what is happening now is better than what happened before. In order to have an EMO, you must be conscious of each stroke, of each moment; once you start comparing (and "losing"), you are somewhere else. If you find yourself going down any of these paths, take a break and start with a fresh cycle.

This is especially necessary for men, who tend to focus so much attention on their future ejaculation that they miss much of what happens in the present. The highest goal is not ejaculation but taking every ounce of pleasure from every stroke. The EMO encompasses all the pleasure that is experienced—starting, possibly, with the very first stroke—not just the squirt at the end. The more you enjoy each stroke, the easier it is to get close to ejaculation. There is no performance anxiety because you are not trying to get anywhere—only to feel.

✒ The Importance of Relaxation ✒

If you want to learn to *give* an orgasm, there are many techniques to learn, but if you want to learn to *receive* one, you need to do as little as possible. The person getting done—the one being rubbed on, the "doee"—needs to be free to put as much attention as feasible on what he or she feels, especially on the stroke that's happening currently. The doee must be focused on the present moment. We have repeatedly stated that the best way to receive an EMO is to be as relaxed as possible. In order to be relaxed, you must not be doing anything.

It takes energy to tense a body part. This is energy that distracts you from focusing on the sensations you feel. Being productive human beings, however, we often find it difficult to relax, and the tensed-up state may seem more natural to us. The common image most people hold of an orgasm is of a man who tenses his body until he ejaculates. Women have been conditioned to imitate this way of having an orgasm. Therefore, it may take some practice and training to learn to relax while a partner pleasures you. Whenever you feel tension in a part of your body, tell yourself to relax. Ask your partner to notice when you tense up and to remind you to relax. Your body knows how to relax, and given a reminder, it usually does. A good way to notice if a partner is tensed is to sense whether his or her anus is tensed or relaxed. You can train your partner to tell you to relax your anus if your partner notices that it's tense. (Your partner need not put a finger inside your anus to check this; the finger just needs to be nearby.)

Relaxing the entire body—avoiding tenseness anywhere, especially in the genital area—allows you to feel the most sensation for the longest time. By contrast, tenseness restricts the flow of blood and oxygen to the nerves and muscles of the genital area; this in turn limits your ability to feel pleasurable sensation. Relaxing also places you in the most receptive state; when you're relaxed, all your energy can be used to feel the sensation rather than to try to produce it yourself or to try to hold your body in a certain position. Some women who have been trained in EMO spread their fingers and toes, while still keeping them relaxed, and allow the sensation of the orgasm to move through their entire bodies and exit through their toes and fingers. Instead of trying to hang on to sensation, they let it flow in and out naturally; this allows even more sensation to enter.

Men in particular have a difficult time remaining relaxed and "at effect" (we use this phrase to refer to a state in which one only receives attention, and does not give attention). They have been conditioned to be aggressive go-getters, to be producers, to take care of business and to prevent others from controlling them. When it is time to lie still, be controlled, receive an orgasm, most men want to help by moving and humping their hips. But they must learn to lie back and be at total effect if they wish to experience the pleasure of an EMO. This goes for women, too. They must lie still and not try to help. The smallest movement in a woman's pelvis makes it more difficult for her partner to keep a finger on her spot.

When people get high with orgasmic sensation, they sometimes hold their breath. This is not good for their orgasm or for their health. We teach our students to breathe normally during orgasm. We don't want them hyperventilating or suffocating. Nor do we want them to perform any kind of breathing exercise, as doing this removes attention from what they feel. They are not giving birth, so special breathing is unnecessary. It is okay to breathe through the mouth, but it is best to breathe through the nose, or through both the nose and mouth. One of the signs of orgasm is an increased breathing rate. This is fine, as long as you do not switch your attention from your genitals to your breathing. We have known many women, and some men, who could experience a very intense orgasm while continuing to breathe quite normally.

⤳ The Push Out ⤳

A method we teach called the "push out" has helped a lot of our students learn to relax. You can do the push out while you are masturbating or while you are getting done.

A sphincter muscle shaped like a figure eight encircles the anus and the vagina (on a woman) or the base of the penis (on a man). This muscle is used in defecating and urinating. When we tense, we contract and "pull up" this muscle. To reverse the tensing and relax, deliberately push out on the muscle, as though you were going to the bathroom. Push out for a few seconds, and then relax the muscle. Be sure to continue breathing normally while you're pushing out. Do this any time you feel yourself starting to tense, such as when sensual stimulation reaches a high intensity, which often provokes tenseness. You might even ask your partner to tell you to push out when he or she feels you beginning to tense. "Push out" and "relax" are two commands that will help you to feel more.

It is a good idea to go to the bathroom before engaging in any kind of sexual experience; this is especially true if you are going to be pushing out. We recommend placing a towel under your buttocks in case of any accidents on the bed. The towel also protects the bedding from normal sexual secretions and any excess lubricant.

You can practice pushing out by inserting a small, clean plastic tube or bottle that has been lubricated into your vagina or anus. Using your sphincter muscles, expel or push out the bottle. You will find this quite easy to do, and it will give you confidence. You can also practice pushing out without a bottle. Then practice pushing out while masturbating.

The first several times you practice pushing out, you may find that your orgasm or your ejaculation is less intense than it was before. This is normal, for when a person is learning a new technique, they often feel awkward or clumsy the first few times, before they become accustomed to the new method. However, if you continue to practice pushing out, you will most assuredly experience more intense and longer orgasms—as all our students have reported.

When a woman gets genitally aroused, her vaginal wall tends to balloon outward. The act of pushing out collapses this balloon; the result is a snugger fit for the penis during intercourse. Pushing out also lengthens the vagina—so the penis is less likely to bang against the cervix—and relaxes the vaginal opening, yielding more pleasure for both partners.

Men who learn to push out as they start to ejaculate—that is, at the point of no return—can intensify their ejaculatory contractions and actually lengthen the entire ejaculatory phase. This results from increased relaxation.

Surrender

We are able to "turn up" the feeling in any part of our body that is touched. (Practicing the touching exercise found in the "Pressures" chapter, later in the book, enhances this ability.) Accordingly, we are each responsible for how much we feel. Phrased another way, we're each responsible for how much we are willing to surrender our nervous system to pleasure.

If we choose to surrender to pleasure, we can turn on any body part at will; we can feel every pore, every nerve ending, every little change in sensation. However, any fear—such as fear of being physically hurt or being taken advantage of—prevents us from surrendering. If we think we owe our partner something in exchange for what they are doing to us, we are unable to surrender fully. If we are angry with the person who is doing us, or if we are angry in general, we are unable to surrender fully. (This is a potential issue for women in particular, many of whom carry unresolved anger toward men for millennia of being treated as second-class citizens. See our book *Extended Massive Orgasm* for a detailed discussion of this matter.) Any doubt that creeps into our minds, whether it is doubt of the person who is giving us pleasure or doubt of our own ability to be pleased, keeps us from surrendering. If we don't sense that the person doing us is in full control of the space or of our nervous system, we are unable to surrender. If we fail to believe that an EMO is possible, we avoid surrendering. Remember that an EMO requires us to surrender to pleasure, rather than to surrender to another person; if we refuse to surrender to pleasure, we are unable to experience the ride of our lives.

Training for the Doee

It is up to you to get your partner to touch you exactly as you want. You will discover this only through thorough exploration of your own body. Then you must communicate your preferences to your partner. Yet, as we said earlier in the chapter, the doee should do as little as possible; this means avoiding having to think or to do much talking and explaining. So how does the doee get his or her partner to touch in the ways that feel best? How does the doee get his or her partner to take control of the space and of the doee's nervous system? This is where communication skills—and a willingness to communicate—come in. You can explain to your partner beforehand how you like to be touched, and where. Using your own hand, you can show your partner how you'd like to be touched. You can touch your partner on the back of his or her hand to demonstrate the amount of pressure you want. You can do your partner first to demonstrate how to control a sensual experience. And, of course, giving your partner a copy of this book beforehand might help. You can also train your partner while he or she is actually doing you.

Some people find the phrase *training your partner* offensive. If you prefer any of the words *teaching, guiding, educating,* or *instructing,* then use those terms instead. The bottom line is that you still must do this—whatever you call it— to get your partner to be the wonderful lover that he or she can be.

"Training from doee," or training for the doee, involves a three-step communication process; the same technique works for men and women. It is designed to yield the most benefit with the fewest number of words. Using this technique helps the doee avoid expending the extra energy involved in giving lengthy explanations, descriptions, justifications, and the like.

The first step is to let your partner know they are doing well. You do this with some form of verbal acknowledgment and approval. The second step is to make a request—ask your partner to do something new or to change what they are doing. As soon as they demonstrate that they are following your request to even a small degree, let them know that they are succeeding by again giving them verbal appreciation; this is step three. (The method is also known as the "sandwich technique": you sandwich your request for a change between two compliments.)

Now go back to step one, and again give your partner further acknowledgment. Only then can you ask for another change. Leave time for at least a breath between approval and request. It is better to say, "Your hand feels great. Will you stroke a little lighter?" than to say, "Your hand feels great *and* would you stroke a little lighter?" We also recommend that you avoid using the word *but* preceding a request. The word *but* has a negating quality; when we hear it, we tend to forget whatever was said immediately beforehand, even if what was said was a compliment.

Keep repeating the three steps until you get your partner to touch you exactly as you want. The following is an example of the training cycle as it could be used by a man who is getting done. "Your hand on my penis feels exquisite. Will you use an up-and-down stroke? That feels wonderful. You have marvelous, soft, yet strong hands. Will you use a long stroke from the base of my penis to the tip? Wow! That feels fantastic. Keep doing that same stroke. Yes! Yes! This is great. You are the best. Will you lighten up a little as you go over the apex and corona? That is even better. You get me so hard. You are so sexy. I think there is a loose pubic hair; will you check and remove it, please? You got it; great! This is the best. You touch me so well."

Note that you can always throw in extra acknowledgments. And remember that the request is always preceded and followed by verbal approval. If you forget to do that, don't fret; just remember to do it next time. To prompt your creativity about what to say when acknowledging your partner, see "Ideas for Communication," in the back of the book.

This technique is great in the bedroom, but it can be used in all facets of life, whenever you want to train someone to do something or want to request a change in behavior. You can train your children to listen to you if you get into agreement with what they *are* doing before telling them what you *want* them to do—that is, if you give them lots of approval before asking for something. If you give your boss some positive feedback before asking for time off or more money, you are more likely to get a favorable response. We don't guarantee that you will get the raise, but everyone likes acknowledgment, so your chances of getting what you want will increase.

Here's an example of how Vera and I have used this technique outside the bedroom. There is a hot tub in our building complex. The temperature had been kept between 102 and 104 degrees. One day, we got in and it was about 97 degrees. We saw the maintenance man who is in charge of the temperature and condition of the tub. We told him what a wonderful job he was doing in keeping the tub clean and well maintained. Then we asked why the temperature had been lowered. He said that a tenant had complained that it was too hot. We asked if he could raise it a few degrees. He said okay, and we thanked him. The next time we got in, it was 100 degrees. We told him that that was better. We said that he was such a good man to look out for everyone's best interests; then we asked if he could please raise the temperature a little. Again he said okay. We told him we appreciated him for that. The next time we used it, the tub was at 103 degrees. He came by, saw us in the tub, and asked if it was hot enough. We thanked him enthusiastically. He was trained.

Acknowledgment, Approval, and Appreciation: More Benefits

Even though you may already have trained your partner in how to touch you just right, it is always a good idea to continue giving acknowledgment any time your partner does something you like, or any time a particular touch feels good. That way, your partner does not have to wonder if he or she is doing it right. Sounds and moans are okay, but since we are capable of language, using words is the best way to communicate approval. You do not have to use eloquent descriptions or wordy statements. A simple "Yes" or "That stroke on my spot feels great" more than suffices.

Some days, you may feel like trying something new, something different from what you usually enjoy. You may normally prefer a light stroke, but on this day, you want to check out how it feels to be touched with a lot of pressure. You can communicate this to your regular partner—either in advance or when your partner is touching you—and he or she probably will be glad to accommodate you. Just be sure to shower your partner with praise before you request any changes, and be as specific with your acknowledgments as you can.

There are three reasons that it is a good idea for the doee to use lots of acknowledgments. First, it removes all doubt in the doer's mind about whether you are enjoying what he or she does. When you withhold approval and appreciation, you actually communicate something; that thing is mystery. When the doee or doer doubts and wonders about their performance, they cannot focus all their attention on the stroke—and they usually assume their performance is unsatisfactory. This negative attitude can turn into anger and antagonism, which in turn can manifest themselves in either loss of turn-on, injury to the genitals, or both. Anger nullifies turn-on, and the result is loss of engorgement and pleasurable sensations. People find it hard to admit that, although they are supposedly doing something pleasurable and wonderful, they actually feel antagonism toward their partners. Rather than admit this negative emotion, they feel guilty about it and go into denial. Denial leads to numbness, and that is when injury can result.

Second, it is beneficial to acknowledge and approve of all the good that is happening because doing so allows you to go higher. We like to compare the act of verbal appreciation to the act of swallowing while eating. You can put only a certain amount of food in your mouth before you have to swallow—that is, if you want to eat more. When you fail to approve of, appreciate, and verbally acknowledge the wonderful sensations and glorious pleasures you experience, you quickly fill up until you are unable to experience more. Just as the simple act of swallowing allows you to eat more, the simple act of acknowledging pleasurable sensations—of symbolically taking them in—allows you to feel more.

Third, it is important to verbally appreciate your partner's actions because the act of talking about what you experience helps to focus you on what is happening and thus helps you to be present with each stroke, in the moment it occurs. Deliberately acknowledging this moment's wonderful feelings prevents your mind from wandering into the past or into the future. It keeps you in the "now," which is where you want to be in order to get the most out of a sensual experience. Acknowledging each other verbally is good for the doer as well as the doee; if both partners verbally acknowledge what is happening, then no one wanders or wonders what the other person is feeling and experiencing.

It is okay to moan and make noise while you are getting off. But the purpose of moaning is to create a pleasant feeling in your throat and vocal area. Do it only if it feels good. The moaning is not meant to impress your partner or to prove how much pleasure you feel. We have known women who, instead of powerfully getting off, pretended to be having a great orgasm by expressing themselves through intense moaning. They put more attention on their noises than on their pleasure. This is confusing to the person doing you, as there is a discrepancy between what your partner senses in you and the energy of the moan. It is also important that any moaning not interfere with verbal communication.

We are so conditioned to avoid talking about sex and to avoid talking during sex that most people at first must make a deliberate effort to communicate while getting done. Most people would rather lie there, say nothing, and let things happen. This is just an old habit; after practicing better communication a few times during sex, it becomes easier to do—effortless, really.

Advice for our female readers: Most men truly want to give the women in their lives as much pleasure as they can. If the woman fails to tell him what she likes, if she fails to tell him where she likes it best, if she fails to tell him exactly how to touch her to give her the most pleasure, he is able to take her only as high as he already knows how to. And for most untrained men, this is not very high. Getting him to read this book will help a lot. Talking to him and telling him your desires will not scare a good man away. Also, give him lots of positive feedback every time he responds to your requests. Many women are looking for a Prince Charming who will wake them with a kiss, sweep them off their feet, and know exactly how to give them that big, wonderful orgasm every time. Prince Charming is only a fairy tale; there is no such person. A woman must expose her appetites, give specific instructions, and exercise lots of patience. By doing this and by appreciating everything he does for you, you create your own prince. Men love to succeed. When you appreciate the way he touches you and let him feel that he is winning with you sexually, he wants to repeat the experience.

As the doee, you want the person doing you to take you for a ride, to notice if you go up or down, and to be aware of what you feel. This will not always be the case. Sometimes your mind may wander, you may stop feeling, and your partner may fail to notice. Don't get upset with your partner or with yourself. Just report that you missed a few strokes. You can ask for a break if you want to talk more or if you think a break would help. This is why talking and acknowledging the good feelings are important. They keep you in present time and give your mind less opportunity to wander. If you are thirsty, don't brave it out. Ask for a drink so you can stop focusing attention on your thirst and put it back on the pleasure of your genitals.

As we mentioned earlier in the chapter, while being done you may find yourself comparing your actual experience to how well you think you should be getting off, or to how memorably you got off another time. Anytime you find yourself comparing, you are in your head; that means you're failing to feel this moment's stroke. If you notice your mind wandering into comparisons—or anywhere else—gently bring your attention back to the stroke at hand. A well-trained doer probably will notice that you've gone away before you notice, but if the doer is less experienced or has gone into his or her own head—which often happens—all you need to do is simply start to feel the stroke again. And, because it bears repeating, appreciating and verbally acknowledging the pleasure you experience in the moment that it happens helps to keep you from going into your head.

We have seen many women students in full orgasm who were oblivious to how much they were getting off. Their bodies were doing great, but their minds failed to notice. Their attention was focused too much in their heads. All they needed to do was to put their attention on their clitorises. With enough practice, the mind catches up to the clitoris and is able to feel each stroke as it happens.

It's also important to learn to notice when you're actually experiencing an EMO—this is something that puzzles some newcomers. The first step in recognizing that you are having an orgasm in a relaxed state is to notice that your genitals, either your clitoris or penis, are feeling more pleasure than any other part of your body. If you put your attention on your genitals, and approve of whatever amount of feeling you experience, your orgasm grows in intensity. You may notice engorgement and muscular contractions in your genitals. You know that the orgasm has become extended, longer than usual, when you can feel pleasurable sensations and contractions for much longer than you have before, when in the usual, tensed-up kind of orgasm. The more approval and attention you focus on your sensations—and the more approval and attention you receive from your partner as he or she peaks you at the right times—the higher the intensity of your orgasm. You know that you're experiencing an EMO when both the duration and the intensity of this new, relaxed orgasm surpasses your old ways of coming and you realize that this is a sensation far superior to any you previously thought possible.

Fantasy

It's great to be done while all of your senses are stimulated in ways that you like—while hearing music you love, smelling fragrances you enjoy, and touching textures that please you, for example. It is also great to have your sixth sense—your conceptual thought—stimulated to add to these pleasurable sensations. Stimulation of your conceptual thought can come in the form of personal fantasy or erotic dialogue.

Fantasy involves using the imagination to create thoughts about something that isn't really happening. You can think about whatever turns you on, whether it is performing a specific sex act with your current partner or doing something or someone entirely imaginary. Our minds link our feelings and thoughts with our physical sensations to determine whether and to what extent something is pleasurable. When you use fantasy to make sensations more intense and pleasurable, you add to the experience in a positive way.

Expressing your fantasy to your partner can make your sensation even better. This includes your partner in what is taking place in your mind. It also allows your partner to play with your fantasy—to embellish it and add to it. While your partner does you, either this time or in the future, he or she can bring up the fantasy, intensifying your experience. However, sometimes a partner might get offended if you talk about a fantasy that involves someone else, whether that someone is a real person or an imaginary lover. If that is the case and you know it in advance, keep the fantasy to yourself.

Fantasy is best used to aid and add to your pleasure. If you indulge in fantasy while taking your attention off the actual stroke, you miss the point. Some people like to watch pornographic videos while having sex. This is fine, as long as you focus on the actual strokes and can stay in communication with your partner. And bear in mind that he or she needs to be in agreement that you'll watch the video.

Some people fantasize a lot, and others hardly at all. Men often fantasize visually, without imagining much of a plot or story line. They might fantasize about a woman they know or have seen, or even about just her leg, breast, butt, or pussy. She might be doing something to them, or they might be doing something to her. I have fantasized about some woman's thigh pressed against my penis—then another woman enters my thoughts and she may sit on my face. These women may or may not have a face, and they do little, if any, talking. Women often indulge in fantasies that have a plot, dialogue, costumes—a whole scene. A woman's fantasy might take place on a train or even in outer space; she meets a guy, exchanges flirtatious glances, and gets to know him. They may or may not even get naked. Women can also have the more basic, doing-the-nasty-with-three-guys-at-once type of fantasy.

We have known gay and lesbian students and fellow researchers who say that they fantasize about the same sex when they are being stroked by someone of the opposite sex. We have known heterosexuals who, when stimulated by a member of the same sex, fantasize about the opposite sex.

Gay men, like straight ones, usually have simpler and more visual fantasies than women, straight or lesbian, do.

Heterosexual women are more likely to fantasize about sexual experiences with another woman than straight men are to fantasize about sex with another man. Straight women also are much more likely to actually allow themselves to be stimulated by a member of the same sex than heterosexual men are. Heterosexual men, in our experience, are more agreeable to being done by another man if a woman is also present. These same men said they did not fantasize about men, and the only way they could allow a man into their fantasies was if he were involved with another woman. Sometimes a man may fantasize that he is a voyeur, watching another man and a woman. No heterosexual man has ever told us that he fantasized about watching two men together. There is simply a bigger taboo in our society against men getting together than there is against women, who can hold hands, touch, and even kiss other women in public without fear of being labeled homosexual. This taboo is so strong that it has invaded our fantasy lives, just as the Oedipal and Electra complexes keep us from fantasizing about sex with our parents. Breaking small taboos and rules can be quite erotic and fun, and fantasy allows us to do this. However, there are a few major societal rules that we are more comfortable upholding even in our fantasies.

You can also talk and fantasize about your partner while he or she is doing you. Your partner is free to respond and even to act out the fantasy. One time, while I was getting done, I remarked that I fantasized about the woman using her leg to get me off. This was just a fantasy; I did not think she would do it. But she got into a position from which she could stroke her leg over my penis. It was very erotic, and I still fantasize about it today. Usually it's more fun to allow a fantasy to remain a fantasy, however, rather than to bring it into reality. Sometimes, however, it is fun to push the envelope a little and to realize a fantasy. You may have a wonderful fantasy and then act it out—only to find out that it was better as a fantasy. This does not have to ruin the fantasy; you can continue to fantasize about someone or something even if the real-life experience was less fun than you had imagined.

Some people like to experiment with S and M, or with dominant and submissive role-playing. As long as nobody gets hurt and everyone is in agreement, it is fine to play these games, which can add a certain eroticism to your normal routine. Talk beforehand about what you would like to happen. You may want to be tied up, handcuffed, blindfolded, whipped, or spanked. Make sure you have decided on a "safe word" before you start; when anyone uses the safe word, it means that he or she really wants to stop. This allows you to say things such as "Stop" or "Don't do that" and not mean it—but the safe word, which might be something as ordinary as "Hello," means that you really do want your partner to stop. These games can be fun to do sometimes, but when you really want to get off—to focus your attention on the intensity of the orgasm—it is better, in our opinion, to get done without the extra distractions of role-playing.

Approaching Ejaculation

When a man is learning to have an EMO, he is learning to get as high as he can without ejaculating. He is training himself to know just how much sensation will take him over the edge. He wants to stay just on this side of ejaculation, at the point where one or two more strokes would send him to the point of no return. The better he can predict when he'll need to stop or take a break, the better he can teach his partner when to stop and what is necessary or most effective for prolonging this phase.

When a man is just on this side of ejaculation, there are a number of ways he can be peaked. If he is quite high but still feels a couple of strokes away from explosion, the doer can simply stop or do a different stroke. If he feels he's right on the verge, his partner can press against the area just under the scrotum, where the ejaculatory duct is located (see FIGURE 5.3, in the preceding chapter). This stops the squirting in midstream; if he's actually caught in the nick of time, he can reload. Squeezing the head of the penis also works, but once the squirting starts, it may be too late for this maneuver.

If he knows it is too late to do anything, he can have his partner extend the ejaculatory phase as long as possible. He can teach his partner to feel his approaching ejaculation, to really focus intention on lengthening it, and to slow down and lighten up the stroke as the ejaculation runs its course.

We have noticed that sometimes, especially with women who are new to getting men off with their hands, at the moment of ejaculation women space out and go into a nonfeeling mode. They may be giddy with excitement because they've accomplished something new, or they may be freaking out at the sight of squirting semen. In any case, the man can continue to acknowledge his good feelings; then he can ask his partner to put her attention back on his orgasm. He can train her in exactly how much to slow down, and he can talk her through the lightening of pressure on his penis to extend the sensations and prolong the ejaculatory phase. The next time she does him, he can remind her to stay with him while he ejaculates. She will learn how he likes it, and he won't always have to remind her and talk her through her excitement.

The ultimate goal is for the doee to totally surrender his or her nervous system to the doer. When you are training your partner and working to keep your partner conscious, obviously you are unable to fully surrender. This is important to remember while you're in training mode. First things first: you have to get your partner trained before you can totally give it up. Then, once the doer has learned to be in control—whether that means staying conscious through the ejaculation phase or at any other stage of the do—the level of your surrender can grow. The fact that the doer got you to the orgasmic or ejaculatory junction demonstrates that they already have taken partial control, and that you have, to some extent, surrendered. Keep acknowledging all the positive things that your partner does, and your partner will learn to put you at total effect, allowing you to totally surrender.

In order to experience EMO, you must make pleasure a priority in your life. You must practice masturbating (as we explained in the prior chapter) and then practice with a partner. You are responsible for training or teaching your partner exactly how you like to be touched and how to take full control of your nervous system. It is easy to control someone who is willing to surrender but almost impossible to control someone who isn't. The extent to which you are willing to surrender is up to you. You have the ability to decide which is most important: feelings like anger or fear that may keep you from surrendering, or your pleasure.

The next chapter explores EMO from the point of view of the person who is giving the orgasm, offering advice on what a doer can do to make an orgasm even better. Then, Chapters 8, 9, and 10 provide more detail about pressures, what the doer can do with the second (or nondoing) hand, and how to bring your partner down.

CHAPTER SEVEN

Whether you are doing a man or a woman, you have to place as much of your attention as possible on your partner in order to produce the maximum orgasm. You must be able to take control of the space of the "do" as well as of your partner's nervous system. We demonstrated in the "Teasing" chapter, earlier, how to get your partner to come toward you with willingness and desire; we now describe how to achieve complete control of the do. Here we delve into techniques for better communication and for peaking your partner. We get into the explicit ways and specific strokes you can use to give your partner a fantastic orgasmic ride. First we explain how to produce an EMO in a woman, and then we explain how to do it to a man. We conclude the chapter with further details on how two people can pleasure each other at the same time.

Giving an EMO

✐ Taking Control ✐

Taking control does not mean that you yell or use force to get your way. Control involves getting into agreement with the situation and proceeding from there. You want your partner to want to surrender; if you get your partner angry with you, you are not in control. The best way to get your partner to a place of surrender is through good communication; this demonstrates that your attention is focused on your partner. Each person requires a somewhat different approach, and each time out with that person may require a different strategy, depending on your partner's mood and willingness to relax and surrender. There is no specific formula; each time you must be prepared to act in accordance with what the circumstances and mood call for—this is what we mean by "getting into agreement with the situation." Sometimes it is best to ask questions, and other times it may be best just to give instructions. Sometimes humor is a valid addition to your communication, and other times using a lot of approval might work best.

We know that some people have a controlling side—an inner "control freak"—which can be a negative attribute. However, giving an EMO is a special situation: if your partner wants to surrender his or her nervous system to you, you must take control. In order to surrender the nervous system, the doee has to surrender *to* something, and the easiest circumstance under which to surrender is when the doee can trust that his or her partner is in full control of the entire experience.

In our private sessions with students, I bring Vera or another woman teacher up to a heightened state and then let the student take my place and continue giving the orgasm. After quite a few sessions, once the student has gotten the knack of the technique and has watched me control the space, we ask the student to start doing the woman from the beginning. We want to see how well the student can control the space—that is, the physical space or area where the "do" takes place. This includes proper pillow positioning, placement of towels and lubrication, and whatever else the doee needs in order to feel that she is cared for. It also involves communicating—telling her where and when she is to lie down, for example—and everything else the student needs to do before giving her an orgasm. We have found that, even after many sessions of watching, some students panic when it's their turn to be in control. In such cases, we take back control from them and give them another chance later, when they usually are more prepared and more ready to take control. Remember that the goal is to have the doee feel taken care of and safe, so that the doee can surrender his or her nervous system. The way one takes control and shows responsibility from the get-go has a great lasting effect. It is very important to make a good first impression, so we insist that our students become experts at this. If they can do it under the pressure of teachers watching and grading them, it becomes much easier when they are in the privacy of their own bedrooms.

When we have a private session with a woman who is learning to receive an EMO, I usually first give Vera or another female teacher an EMO while the student watches. I focus attention both on the teacher's orgasm and on the student. I instruct the student to feel as much of the orgasm in her own body as she can, even though she has not yet been touched. I suggest that the student "feel her own pussy." When it is the student's turn to receive an orgasm, sometimes I get into position first and have the student lie down perpendicular to me; other times, I have the student lie down while I investigate her genitals from a standing position, sensually touching her feet or legs, and then get into the sitting position for doing. We make sure her legs are spread apart and that her outer leg comfortably rests on a pillow. It's fun to start each session a little differently. It keeps the woman wondering what you will do next and promotes curiosity and creativity from the very beginning.

The person who does the "doing" permits the doee to relax and give up control if the doer has a confident attitude and demonstrates this confidence through his or her very presence. This does not mean doers should brag about how great they are; they simply need to feel confidence in themselves and let this confidence shine out. Avoid saying self-deprecating things such as "I don't know what I'm doing" or "This is the first time I've ever done this." Avoid saying "Oops" or "Whoops" if you think you've made a mistake; you want the doee to feel that you are in control, confident that you know what you are up to and that everything you do is deliberate. If you move off the doee's spot by accident or by spacing out, take responsibility as soon as possible, saying, for example, that you've deliberately moved off the spot in order to peak or bring down your partner. Act like everything that happens is deliberate, that you planned it that way.

As the doer, you may find that your partner does or says little things that seem innocuous but actually are attempts to resist being controlled. Your partner may start touching or stroking your arm or leg during the do. There is nothing wrong with allowing the doee to touch you—except when it feels like an attempt to undermine your control or it is done in a way that makes you feel at all strange or suspicious. If the doee surprises you by starting to touch you during the do, you can ask the doee to take his or her hand away. Tell the doee that you'll let them touch you if they ask nicely and if you think it will get them to feel more. Otherwise, refuse to let them get away with it, as they may continue to probe to see how much control they can take back. Trust your own integrity; only allow what feels good and right to you.

If you have learned to be great at teasing, that makes the rest of "doing" that much easier. If you can raise your partner to a heightened state of tumescence before actually stroking their spot, you have already gotten them. Enthusiasm is contagious, and if you are enthusiastic about the experience, your partner will probably become more eager. Enthusiasm can be demonstrated by loving what you are doing and communicating how thrilled you are. Each time out is a unique experience, and when you can relate to your partner (especially a long-term partner) the freshness and novelty of this new adventure, you only help whet their appetite. You have learned, if you have read the previous chapters, how to tease, how to lubricate, and how to position your hands. Now it is time to take your partner for a ride of intense orgasm.

Training to Do

When you first learn how to best stimulate your partner—whether your partner is a man or a woman—it is a good idea to ask them lots of questions about what they like. Initiate a conversation beforehand to find out all you can about what your partner likes and doesn't like, where they would like it, and where and how they would prefer that you begin. (As we said in the prior chapter, this is why it's important for the doee to first explore his or her own body; armed with this self-knowledge, doees can respond thoroughly to their partners' questions and volunteer any information that would make the experience more fun. Doees should consider actually demonstrating to their partners, using their own hands, where and how they like to be touched.)

Once you begin stimulating your partner, it is best to keep questions simple and easy to answer. The person who is stimulated feels the most when they are relaxed and can put as much attention as possible on their pleasurable sensations. You want to avoid requiring them to think too much or to do anything that takes away from what they feel. We recommend that you pose only questions that can be answered with a simple "yes" or "no." Now is not the time for essay questions or "why" questions. Avoid questions such as "How does this feel?" Also, ask only questions whose yes-or-no answers won't cause either partner to "lose." This means that questions such as "Does this feel good?" or "Do you like this stroke?" are prohibited; if the doee responds with a no, the person asking the question loses. Or the doee might decide to lie rather than hurt the doer's feelings. Therefore, because the truth in sex will set you free and lies will dampen the orgasm, avoid creating an environment that permits lying.

However, there are lots of questions you *can* ask, such as "Would you like more pressure? Would you like less pressure? Would you like it more to the left? More to the right? More under the hood? Would you like a shorter stroke just on the apex?" The more curious and attentive you are, the more questions that will occur to you.

Let's say you've asked, "Would you like it more to the left?" If your partner says yes, immediately move your finger or hand to the left, but only in a small increment. Then repeat the question; as long as your partner answers yes, keep moving to the left, and keep asking until your partner says no. You can then ask if your partner would like it more to the right; if your partner says no, you know you are at the right place.

EXERCISE Some people who are new to talking during a sensual experience find it helpful to practice their communication skills while touching a body part other than the genitals. People have a lot of "charge" on their private parts, and it can be difficult to learn to talk when you begin by rubbing the genitals right away.

For this exercise, two people decide who will be the doer and who will be the doee. Then they agree on a specific area of the doee's body that the doer will touch. This body part can be an inner thigh, the belly, or anywhere else that the two partners agree upon. The person getting stroked lies down in a comfortable position. The person stroking sits at the doee's side and, before anything is done, communicates everything he or she will do. The doer can practice controlling the space by keeping the doee informed and relaxed about any noises (such as a ringing phone) or other extraneous events that may occur.

Before the doer puts a hand on the doee, the doer first defines the area that they will rub. Let's say they've agreed on the inner thigh; the doer can define the area to be rubbed as the space from the knee to right below the pubic-hair line. Now the doer puts a hand on the area and begins rubbing with a steady, reliable stroke. The specific stroke the doer uses does not matter, but the doer must repeat the same stroke, using the same speed and pressure.

Now the doer begins asking questions. "Would you like it faster, slower, harder, lighter, with the palm of the hand, with the back of the fingernails?"—whatever the doer can think of to ask. All the doee has to do is answer yes or no. If the answer is yes, the doer makes the requested change in small increments. If the doee is unsure what they want, they can just answer no till they are sure.

After getting comfortable with a less-charged body part, the doer can move to stroking the genitals, if both partners agree, keeping the same communication structure.

Once you have trained and communicated with the same partner over a number of sessions, you no longer will have to ask the same questions all the time. When you reach this level, you can focus more attention on your partner and use skilled communication to help you control the orgasm. The kinds of communication you can use at this stage include giving lots of approval; telling them how much fun it is to touch them, that they are coming wonderfully, that you can feel their orgasm; and telling them how beautiful and sexy they are (especially if the doee is a woman). You can also issue commands and requests: "Relax!" "Take it higher!" "Let's take it up." "Give me more!" When giving a command or request, it is important that you have strong intentions to accompany the words. And be sure to acknowledge your partner as soon as he or she goes in the requested direction. You can also say things such as, "I've got you now; there is no escape!" The word *yes* can be used in either the doer or doee position and is always a win. See "Ideas for Communication," in the back of the book, for more things to say.

After going through initial training, people giving an orgasm can put more energy into feeling the pleasure in their own bodies. When a woman who is stimulating someone feels her own pussy and clitoris, especially in relation to her partner's genitals, she adds to both partners' pleasure. Learning to feel and to take pleasure while touching your partner is one of the most important aspects of producing a great orgasm.

⚞ Doing a Woman ⚟

When you start a "do date" or session, the important things to remember are to take control, communicate what you are up to, keep your attention on the woman, and, most important, have fun. We have had students who were so preoccupied with getting the techniques right that they forgot to really enjoy what was taking place. That is why it is a good idea to first practice the techniques on a pencil, as we discussed in Chapter 4, and to practice your communication skills on less charged body parts, so that when you get your hands on a woman's genitals you don't freeze up and forget to enjoy yourself.

You take control by making sure everything is just right and presenting an air of confidence. Check that you have the pillows where you want them and that the towels, lubricant, and drinks are easily accessible. Play music that she likes, and make sure the phone won't disturb you. Ensure that the entire environment is up to your standards. Let her know where you want her to lie down and where you will position yourself.

Her clitoris will be thirsting for your touch. You can tease her by almost starting, moving your finger closer and closer to her clitoris, and then withdrawing. By the time you are no longer able to resist touching her spot, she will be seeking out your finger with her clitoris. Upon touching her there, let her know how good it feels, that you are home now and that you have her where you want her. You don't have to use these exact words; choose whatever feels appropriate for you and for the situation.

THE SPOT ↦ It is usually best to reach her spot—that is, the most sensitive spot on her clitoris—with the first stroke. In most women, this is the upper left quadrant (that is, on *her* left side) of the clitoral head. You can find it by imagining that the clitoral head is the face of a clock. From your perspective, looking at the clitoral head straight on, find the spot that corresponds to 1:30 on the clock (see FIGURE 3.1, earlier in the book).

It is not written in stone that a woman's spot is located here. In some women, it could be on the upper right side or toward the middle. However, both on our own and collectively, we have done hundreds of women, and so far we have found that all of them are especially responsive when stimulated on the upper left quadrant. We have noticed on the Internet that a few women claim to be more sensitive on the upper right side and we find this argument plausible, too. The entire clitoral glans is richly innervated, and each person has a slightly different arrangement. But we believe that choosing the upper left quadrant works in over 99 percent of women; unless she vigorously asserts that she prefers another spot, you can feel safe choosing that zone.

Whatever stroke you use, it is best to be confident—never tentative—with your touch. It is better not to touch at all than to be hesitant or unsure. The doee can feel tentativeness right away; this causes her to lose confidence in your lead, which makes surrender that much more elusive. You may not always know what you are doing, but if you do it with an air of confidence, then confidence is what your partner feels, too. This goes for doing men as well as women.

It is essential that people who wish to give EMOs, especially to women, keep their hands and nails in tiptop condition. One sharp nail can ruin a potentially wonderful sexual experience. Keep all your nails short and smooth. If you have calluses on you fingertips, make sure that they are smoothed out. Use hand lotion as often as necessary to keep your hands soft and smooth.

THE SHORT STROKE ✐ We recommend a short up-and-down stroke on the spot on her clitoral head. By "short stroke," we mean a movement of a few millimeters or about one-sixteenth of an inch—or even shorter. We believe a short stroke is best because it allows you to remain on the spot at all times during the stroke. With a longer stroke, you may touch the spot for a part of the stroke, but then you move to other areas of the clitoris or even off the clitoris entirely. The longer stroke, however, may be more pleasurable to a woman who is new to direct clitoral stimulation. In this case, it is better simply to give her fewer strokes than to move off her sweet spot via long strokes. Deliberately giving her long strokes is also okay on occasion, although it's not a preference you want to encourage in her, and therefore long strokes probably are not the best way to begin.

For the basic stroke, slide your finger up and down over the clitoris, without moving the clitoris itself. The pressure and speed of the stroke depend on what feels best at the time. This is where careful communication and focusing your attention on your partner enter the picture. By asking her directly and by "feeling" or sensing her, you tune into what she needs and wants—you sense what will increase her trust in your ability to give her pleasure and therefore will bring her closer to surrender. Sometimes what is called for is a really quick stroke with the tip of your finger, and other times it is a slow stroke that barely moves. It is usually best not to start with very firm pressure: it's easier to add more pressure later, if desired, and you don't want your partner to retreat because you used too much pressure at first. A light to medium pressure is usually a safe bet.

When you anchor the clitoris with your thumb, it makes it easier to stay on the spot and stops the clitoris from playing hide-and-seek with you. You can stroke with the tip of either the index or the middle finger, depending on what feels better in the specific position you're in and how much practice you have with either finger. You may have to hook your stroking finger under the clitoral hood when you first begin—particularly if you are right-handed— even though you are pulling back the hood. Hooking the stroking finger allows it to reach her spot and positions the finger at a good angle (FIGURE 7.1). Left-handed doers may have to hook their finger, too, but they are at a more natural angle (FIGURE 7.2). Refer to the "Positions" chapter if you need a refresher on how to position your hands.

To take someone up, it is best to use a stroke that is dependable and reliable. That means a stroke

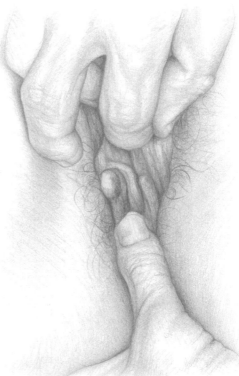

FIGURE 7.1
Right-handed doing position showing how to hook the index finger under the hood to get to the clitoris

FIGURE 7.2
Left-handed doing position with index finger on upper left side of the clitoris

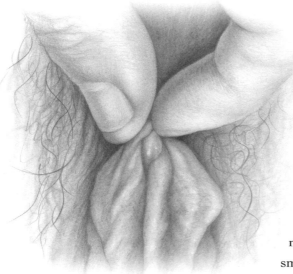

that you do over and over, as long as it feels good. This allows her to surrender to the stroke and not wonder when the next stroke will happen or where it will be. Once she does surrender, it is possible to use a more random stroke.

Continue with the same steady stroke to take her up to the first peak. Feel your finger moving up and down on that small area of her clitoris. As long as the sensation keeps feeling better, continue to stroke. Let her know how good it feels to you, and report any signs of orgasm you observe in her. Recall that the physical manifestations of EMO include phenomena that most people are used to identifying merely as signs of sexual stimulation; the difference is that a fully relaxed, surrendered, tuned-in doee is focused on feeling intense, orgasmic pleasure from the very first stroke. (How to recognize an EMO is described in detail in the preceding chapter, "Receiving an EMO." Become familiar with the signs of orgasm so you can describe them accurately to your partner when they're happening to her.) The clitoris might be getting engorged and harder. Color changes might be occurring all over her vulva, including her labia and clitoris. She may experience flushing—that is, reddening—on her face and neck. She may sweat, and ejaculatory fluid may ooze from her introitus, but probably not on the first peak. Many women who have trained and are advanced in their ability to reach orgasm have strong contractions in their abdomens; we call this "abdominal ridging." If she likes to play with fantasy, you can tell her one that she will enjoy. Let her know when the sensation continues to climb.

PEAKING When you, the doer, first start to think that the next stroke won't be quite as exquisite as the last one, or when you start to wonder if she is going up anymore, it is time to deliberately take the orgasm down a notch or two. This technique is called *peaking*. The way to take the orgasm down, or to end the peak, is to change the stroke. You can stop touching her altogether for a split second or indefinitely. You can change the speed, pressure, or location of the stroke. You can give her a few firm strokes. Any of the above will bring her down. Let her know that you are peaking her or taking her down, and continue talking even if you bring her down for only a short time. By deliberately taking her down before she's ready to come down or before she's noticed that she's had enough, you enable her to want more.

Then you can start a new cycle, taking her up to a new peak. Let her know that you are going to take her back up. You can go back to using the same stroke that you used before, or you can use another one—a faster or a slower stroke, a firmer or a lighter stroke. There is no formula; do what feels best to your hand at the time. You can ask your partner what she wants and then do what she suggests. If you do as she requests and it does not feel as good as before or fails to evoke the response you believe she could feel, thank her for her input and let her know that you will change the stroke again. Ultimately, you have to learn to trust yourself and go with what you feel is best.

The length of the break between each peak is not predetermined; it varies throughout the session. Sometimes you may want to quench your thirst or talk about what just happened. Other times you may want to dip her for just a split second and take her right back up with the same stroke. Basically, the longer the break between peaks, the farther down she comes. Women who are new to this kind of experience usually require more time between peaks and lots of talking about what they've experienced. A woman who can get off easily and has experienced EMOs requires a much shorter break and is ready to go back up right away. Again, this is not written in stone; it's only a general guideline.

The length of each peak also varies. Some peaks last for only one or two strokes, and others go on for minutes. Again, with women who are new to this experience, the length of the peak tends to be on the short side. They are unused to feeling so much sensation directly on their clitorises, and their attention span for pleasure is still undeveloped. It is better to give them three strokes that they feel completely than one hundred strokes of which they feel only 20 percent. The goal is to have them feel every stroke and for you to enjoy every stroke you give them.

If you begin with short peaks, you will have more of her attention. She will feel more, and you can then gradually lengthen the peaks. Some women are naturals and can have long peaks the first time out. This is rather unusual, but it is a reason to stay awake and notice how many strokes in a row she can feel. If a woman practices direct clitoral stimulation while masturbating, she can feel more, and feel it longer, when someone else stimulates her.

CLITORAL SIZE Once she is getting off well and is fully engorged, her clitoris usually bulges out from its hood. Although the most sensitive spot in most women remains the upper left quadrant, the entire clitoris is more sensitive now, and touching it all over can bring her up.

Some women have small clitorises that may not bulge out. If this is the case, you still should be able to feel the clitoris: because it is engorged, it feels like a hard little pellet under your fingertip. Finding the "sweet spot" on a small clitoris presents a challenge, especially if you have large fingers; however, a small clitoris probably has a higher concentration of nerve endings all over it. You can still use a short stroke on the approximate upper left quadrant of a small clitoris; the stroke probably will include more of the rest of the clitoris as well. In Betty Dodson's book *Sex for One, the Joy of Self-Loving*, she has included illustrations of a number of different shapes and sizes of clitorises.

In most women with average-size clitorises that are engorged, you can easily distinguish among the different areas on the clitoris. She already knows that you know where her spot is, so she can relax and surrender to whatever you are doing. To illustrate what we mean, we like to use a base-ball analogy. (If you are not a sports fan, Vera says to skip this analogy.) A great pitcher can throw a baseball over any specific part of home plate. The umpire knows this and calls as strikes all fairly close pitches, even if they are off the plate. The batter knows this, too, and swings at anything close to the plate. Bottom line: the pitcher owns home plate, and everyone knows it. Likewise, a woman who knows that you know her spot—that you own her spot—will surrender her whole clitoris. An untrained woman who thinks you don't know where it is will refuse to surrender at all. Remember that she is not really surrendering to the doer, but to her own greater pleasure. Consequently, a trained woman can surrender, at least to some extent, to even someone who lacks confidence and is inexperienced at producing an EMO. She can have a great orgasm no matter who is doing it. Of course, a confident, trained doer and an accepting, trained doee is the best combina-tion for a great orgasm.

Once the clitoris is fully exposed from its hood, you do not have to con-tinue to pull back on the hood and anchor the clitoris with your thumb. Many women like the feeling of a thumb against the shaft of their clitoris and this position does help keep the clitoris from slipping away, so it may be a good idea to keep the thumb there; it just is less necessary. When the clitoris is exposed, it also becomes less necessary to hook your stroking finger under the hood; you can easily reach any spot. Once the whole clitoris is available, you can create a variety of strokes. You can move about the clitoris at will. Try a few strokes on the right side, some in the middle, a few on the bottom, and then a few back on her spot. As long as you have the intention of taking her up, you'll do so.

DANCING ON THE CLITORIS AND OTHER STROKES A fun way to do a woman is to "dance" on her clitoris. In rhythm to the beat of the music playing, or in a variation on it, let your finger dance on the clitoral head like someone dancing on a dance floor. Most music has repeating patterns; following these, you can return to her spot at regular intervals. You can also peak her to the music; pause in your stroking to coincide with pauses in the music.

For a time, follow the beat of the music; then, when your partner is expecting you to keep sticking with the beat, surprise her with something else—bring her down a little and then take her back up higher, getting into the pattern again. Surprise always brings a doee down at first, so when you use surprise, use it deliberately. It is always a good idea to occasionally go back to her spot to let her know that you have not forgotten where it is and to take her up with optimal ease and speed. We have known people who have made special "doing tapes," on which they chose music to create several choreographed dances on a clitoris. This is just another way to have fun and to be playful while producing a great orgasm.

You can play with a variety of other strokes, too. You can use circular motions around the whole clitoris, or small circles in a specific zone such as the upper left quadrant. You can move back and forth around the upper circumference of the clitoris. You can stroke both sides of the clitoris at once, using your index and middle fingers.

One stroke (very similar to the basic stroke) is an up-and-down motion that moves the part of the clitoris directly below the finger. The finger is still moving up and down, but it is not really sliding along the clitoris; rather, the clitoris is doing the moving. You can also rub across the clitoris from left to right and back again. You can use your thumb directly on the clitoris and move it in any direction that feels great. In the chapter titled "Pressures," later in the book, we offer options for using your second hand to add to the pleasure. You can create your own strokes and even make up your own names for them. Do whatever feels good, as long as you experience pleasure and fun in doing it.

The clitoris may grow hard and engorged during the orgasm; at other times, it becomes less engorged and softer. These usually indicate changing levels of intensity, but the sensation in your finger is the best indicator of whether she is going up or down. It would be nice if there were a light-bulb that got brighter when a woman went up and dimmer when she went down, but in reality you have to pay attention to all the signs, especially the sensation in your finger and the way your body feels. Her clitoris could be fully engorged and hard, and yet, as we have pointed out, she may not be consciously aware of it or how good it feels.

To produce a great orgasm, the only stroke you *have* to use is the short up-and-down stroke directly on her spot. A woman can get off for an hour or more and be totally gratified if you use this surefire and reliable stroke. Other fine and fancy strokes are fun to do and can add variety to your techniques, but it is most important that you master the basic stroke before you diverge into other ones. It is also best to continue with this reliable stroke until she can take lots of pleasure from it. Get her to really feel each stroke on her clitoris, both the up stroke and the down stroke. Once she can come easily with this simple, yet exquisite, stroke, you can add whatever strokes you like.

STAYING IN CONTROL ❧ As we discussed in detail in the chapter "Receiving an EMO," it is vitally important that the doee verbally acknowledge all pleasurable sensations. This is especially important for a woman who is training to have an EMO. We often "threaten" a woman who fails to verbally acknowledge her pleasure with the cessation of her session. If she continues to refuse to talk about her pleasure, we quit the session. It does no good to threaten someone and then fail to follow through on your threat. We may give her a couple of opportunities to "win," but if she continues to resist, we must end the session.

This is a technique that any doer, man or woman, can use to maintain control. You can warn your partner that you will quit doing them if they demonstrate any kind of resistance. They might thrust their pelvis, make nasty comments, fail to acknowledge, or just avoid feeling. Do not make idle threats, and use this method only if you feel that you want to stop. If you don't feel like stopping, don't bring it up. (Bear in mind that for this to work, the doee must be aware of the benefits of acknowledgment and must be in agreement that he or she wants to acknowledge more. If your partner is new to these techniques, ask him or her to read the "Receiving an EMO" chapter.) Remember to reward your partner with positive feedback for any attempt to follow your instructions. And setting a good example by acknowledging and appreciating your partner is another excellent way to get your partner to acknowledge more.

Finally, remember that your partner is a whole person; she is more than just her genitals. Learn to talk easily and to express whatever you are feeling in a loving way. As we have consistently stated, the goal is to have fun, not to see how big an orgasm you can create. The big, wonderful orgasm is a byproduct of how much fun you have. It is probably better to go on a short, fantastic ride than on a long one that is intermittently hot and cold. The ride up can last anywhere from one stroke to hours. It depends on the level of orgasm the doee has trained to receive as well as the time available and both partners' specific goals and desires.

The information provided here is only part of the do. In the following chapters, we describe pressures, what you can do with your second hand, and how to bring your partner down in the most pleasurable way.

✒ Doing a Man ✒

Although men and women have similar nervous and circulatory systems and most of their body parts have a homologous part in the opposite sex, there are still some basic differences. Men's genitals and their most sensitive areas are right out there; you do not have to go hunting or digging for them. By contrast, the most difficult aspects of doing a woman are finding her clitoris, getting on her spot, and staying on it. When doing a man, you encounter none of these problems. However, men do have an ejaculatory response that is different from women's orgasmic response: with men, once the expulsion phase begins, it is difficult to go back. The trick in giving a man an EMO is getting as close as you can to this expulsion without actually triggering it.

Men are more used to having their penises touched than women are to receiving direct clitoral stimulation; therefore, a man's peak, even the first time out, tends to be longer than a woman's. The problem is that most men are used to being stimulated fast and hard. They are tensed rather than relaxed; their goal is ejaculation rather than sensual pleasure. They miss probably 80 percent of each stroke. Here's a good analogy: place your two index fingers against each other, in parallel (see FIGURES 7.3A AND 7.3B). Notice how little you feel when you rub them together rapidly. Now contrast that sensation with how you feel when you move them slowly, over a period of several seconds.

As with a woman, when you're taking a man on an intense orgasmic ride, it is important to demonstrate that you are in charge and are responsible for the whole sensual experience. Men tend to want to be in control and may resist being "at pleasurable effect" (in other words, being the recipient rather than the giver of attention). This resistance is easily overcome, and if the doer shows that she is in charge, knows what to do, and takes full responsibility, he will surrender. If he notices that the doer is timid or tentative, he will avoid surrendering and will try to take back

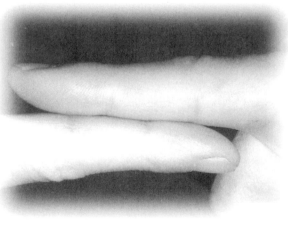

FIGURE 7.3A
Alignment of the two fingers to feel the difference between a slow and fast stroke

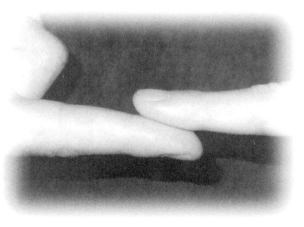

FIGURE 7.3B
Direction of movement from Figure 7.3A

control. The doer demonstrates control by communicating what she will do, what she wants him to do, and how much pleasure she gets from doing him. She takes responsibility for setting up the space, including all necessary paraphernalia and drinks. Any time he begins to tense up or to do something that interferes with what she wants, she immediately lets him know. Once a woman has her hands on a man's penis and is touching him for her own pleasure, he will not want to resist. Some men may start thrusting their hips or trying to help her, but if she lets him know with confidence how she wants him to behave, he will cooperate.

Quite a few women confess to a lack of confidence when it comes to rubbing pleasurably on a man's penis and genitals. Some may have had a negative experience in the past, and others may have little or no experience. Others, hopefully a minority, may be fibbing, pretending to a lack of confidence as an excuse to not have to play with a man's private parts.

Confidence can be easily gained in just one or a few winning encounters. Men are really easy; as long as you touch your man for your own pleasure and act with an air of confidence, things go smoothly. That means you do best if you take charge and do not bring up your fears and doubts when it is time to touch him. By studying the material on male anatomy and teasing, earlier in the book, and the rest of this chapter, you will absorb more than enough information to help you feel confident. Additionally, a number of exercises are presented in the "Pressures" chapter, later, that are beneficial in learning how to touch a man. When you do touch him, touch him with enthusiasm and full knowledge that you are a sexually powerful woman. When his penis is hard and throbbing in your hand, it is yours to do with as you please. You own it, and you know what you are up to. Don't let him think that you don't know what you are doing. Make him think that you were born to have fun with it.

THE STROKES   We have already described teasing, the application of lubricant, and the positioning of your hands. Although the short up-and-down stroke is best on a clitoris, the long stroke is the most reliable for the penis. The apex is the most sensitive area on the penis, but the entire shaft contains a lot of nerve endings. There are a lot of different and wonderful strokes that you can do to a penis. You want to take as much enjoyment from your hands as is possible at all times. In order to bring him up, you want to use a steady, reliable stroke that he can depend upon. Once you find a stroke that feels good to your hand, keep doing it over and over again. This way, he can rely on what you're doing and can surrender to your touch.

As we have indicated, different men prefer different pressures. It is usually good to begin with a fairly firm and sure grip. Don't forget to feel the sensation in your hand when you stroke the shaft and the head; feel your hand both on the way up and on the way down. By talking with him beforehand, or by watching him masturbate, you can learn some things he might enjoy.

Because of the sensitivity around the apex and the head of the penis, it usually is a good idea to lighten the stroke as you reach this area. Then, when you stroke back down the shaft, you can use additional pressure. As long as the stroke is steady and repetitive, you allow him to surrender to that stroke and to go higher. Allow your hand to glide easily along the shaft and up to the corona and head. Feel the texture of his penis against your fingertips. As soon as you change the stroke, you're peaking him and taking him downward. As long as you do that deliberately—and you let him know that you did it deliberately—you stay in control. If he thinks that you either spaced out or don't know what you're doing, he can't surrender.

Here's one of the best strokes: Hold the penis in your hand with your fingertips positioned up and down along the

FIGURE 7.4
Full contact stroke on penis, fingertips along the urethra

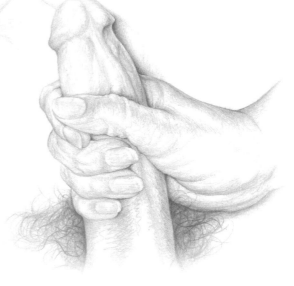

underside of the penis (again, the underside of the penis is the side that's visible when the penis is erect and is pressed against the scrotum when the penis is flaccid). Your thumb is also engaged with stroking the penis, as your whole hand is against the shaft. Get as much surface contact between your hand and the penis as possible (FIGURE 7.4). Use a sort of milking motion with your hand on the way up. Feel the stroke in both directions. Feel every nuance and gradation on the surface of his penis. Feel how hard it can get in your hand. Feel the throbbing and contractions of his penis, and let him know how good that makes you feel. Take him as high as you want him to go without getting to the point of no return. Then deliberately back him off from this height or peak. Let him know what you are doing.

You can tell that a man is having an EMO when he is in a relaxed state, each stroke on his penis and genital area feels sensational, and his penis and pelvic area are contracting involuntarily. The intensity keeps building with each peak, and seminal fluid may ooze out of the urethral opening. Take a break for however long feels right. You are in control, and you have to trust your feelings and intuitions. You may want to sip a drink or offer a sip to your partner. Start again when you feel so inclined. The longer you wait between peaks, the farther down he will go, but men can get back up really fast when you have true intention. You may want to skip just a stroke or two and then start again. If he is quite high and close to the edge, you may be able to give him only a few strokes before he is right back up there again. You can do this pattern—a short break followed by a brief period of stroking—over and over to get him really high and tumesced.

A man can really enjoy it if you just hold his member in your hand and really feel it. You can play with different pressures (see the "Pressures" chapter for some ideas). Caress him with affection. The stroke that feels best to you will feel best to him. You can take his penis in your full hand as if you were going to squeeze it, and then twist your hand back and forth around it. Do this anywhere on his penis that feels good, from the bottom of the shaft to the head.

Another option is to do the up-and-down stroke, but to add the twist once you reach the top—feeling the entire head and apex with that extra circular motion of your hand—and return to the straight stroke on the way down. As long as you repeat the same stroke, he will go higher and higher, until you want to take him down a little by changing it. If you keep changing the stroke on him, he has a more difficult time surrendering and going higher.

After bringing a man up with a steady stroke and deliberately peaking him, you can bring him back up with either the same or a different stroke. You can use one finger just on the apex (which is illustrated in FIGURE 3.11, earlier in the book), rubbing up and down. The speed can be quick or slow, but use the same speed until you decide to switch, and then stay in communication so he knows that you are being deliberate. Make sure you have enough lubricant on your hand, and use less pressure when you're directly on the apex. Some women like to use their thumb to stroke the apex, with the rest of their fingers on the opposite side of the penis. You can also use a full-hand stroke; when you reach the base of his penis, firmly press your hand against his abdomen.

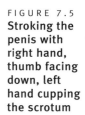

FIGURE 7.5
Stroking the penis with right hand, thumb facing down, left hand cupping the scrotum

Turn your hand so that now your thumb is facing downward instead of upward (FIGURE 7.5). Grasp the penis, using as much surface area of your hand as you can. Using the same motion as when your thumb was pointing upward, stroke from the bottom of the shaft to the head and back down again, pressing into his abdomen if you like. As long as the stroke feels good to your hand and the motion is steady and reliable, he can go higher and higher.

You can use both hands to stroke his penis. Place both hands in contact with it and stroke up and down with the hands together (FIGURE 7.6). You can also do a one-direction stroke: one hand stays on the penis at all times while you stroke up and over the head; then remove that hand and bring it back down to the base of the penis while the other hand strokes up along the shaft, goes over the head, is removed, and is placed back at the base. You can add the twist if you like. In this stroke, the hands go in only one direction, upward, but there is continual stimulation, as the second hand starts its ascent while the first one ends it, and vice versa.

Then there is the "gearshift" stroke: you move the engorged penis around and pull it away from the body at the same time. You can take it as far to the left and the right, as far backward and forward, as it will pleasurably go (FIGURE 7.7). Some men may be afraid of having their penis pulled and moved very far; therefore, move it in small increments at first, until you know how much motion he wants. This stroke works best when the penis is fully engorged and hard.

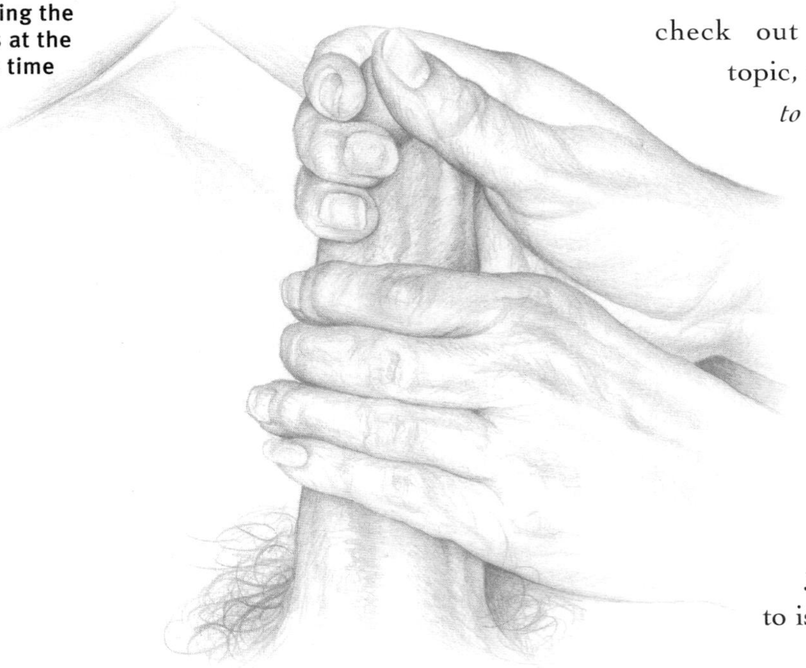

FIGURE 7.6
Two hands stroking the penis at the same time

For more strokes to pleasure the penis, check out other books on the topic, such as Lou Paget's *How to Be a Great Lover*—or create your own wonderful strokes.

TO EJACULATE OR NOT You do not have to bring a man to ejaculation every time you do him. However, *knowing* that you could if you wanted to is a great addition to your

repertoire—it adds to your confidence and, accordingly, to his
pleasure. There are a number
of reasons to refrain from
bringing a man to ejacu-
lation. One could be
that he does not
wish to ejaculate
but rather wants to
experience orgas-
mic pleasure with
peaks. This way is
popular with men
who have studied
tantric sex. Or you may want to play
with his penis with your hands for some time and
then use it for intercourse. You are saving his seed so that you
both will enjoy his ride inside you. Third, perhaps you have done him for a
while and you simply don't feel like doing it anymore. Only touch your partner when and for as long as you want to, and communicate to him when you
have had enough. Some women rub their partner's penis for as long as it is
enjoyable to them, and then watch him finish himself off.

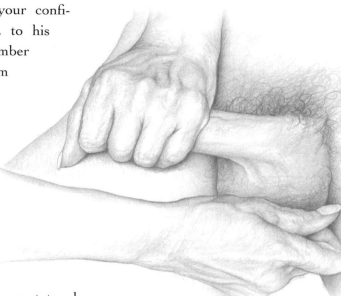

FIGURE 7.7
**The "gearshift"
stroke with
pulling of the
scrotum**

Some men are easier to get off than others. Some men (usually young
and "undercomed"—i.e., they haven't had much sex) start squirting on
the first stroke or even while you are undressing them. Other men may
take a long time. Men who have drunk a lot of alcohol might get what is
called a "whiskey hard-on," or what is technically called a priapism: they
stay hard but are unable to get off. Nonetheless, almost every healthy
man can get off. We have talked to prostitutes who said they had over a
99 percent rate of effectiveness in getting a man off by hand. These
women were not especially beautiful. They had total confidence and did
not spend any time thinking about failing or doubting. They also were

interested in quickly getting a man off, as opposed to seeing how long they could extend his orgasm.

Some men have circulation problems and other medical conditions that prevent their penises from getting erect; they are advised to see a doctor or therapist. It is still possible to have fun with a penis that is flaccid or has difficulty getting erect. The nerve endings are still there, and the soft skin of the penis can be sensually touched and enjoyed. We have known a number of men who thought they were impotent. However, with loving attention from a person who enjoyed touching them without any expectations, they were pleasantly surprised to find that their penises got engorged.

It is not much more difficult to give a man a long orgasm than it is to make him ejaculate. You just have to be aware of how close you are to the edge and get as close to it as possible without falling over it. Some women new to doing men may be thrilled by getting their partners to the edge and then going over it as soon as they can. This is fine, but if you want to become an expert or connoisseur of the male orgasm and of orgasm in general, there is a whole world of pleasure waiting for you.

Most men masturbate, and most ejaculate when they do. You can arrange to watch your partner as he does himself, to see what kinds of strokes he likes to use. Some men may be embarrassed to let someone watch, but when approached seductively, they will probably relent. Bear in mind that men typically use a hard and fast stroke on themselves in order to release tension and tumescence as quickly as possible. You need not emulate exactly how your man touches himself; instead, be choosy about what you want to use from your observations of him.

When a woman gets frustrated and angry with her partner, she nullifies her biggest trump card, which is her turn-on. She must not get angry with him in a do, because it will lead to a fight instead of a great orgasm. She also has to touch for her own pleasure: if she doesn't find it fun to rub hard and fast, it's best that she not pretend she does like it. The slow and light stroke ultimately feels better to the man, too. (If she enjoys rubbing hard or fast, that is OK, too, only she's best served to train him to really enjoy the sensuality of the slow, light touch.) Time, patience, and practice will help both partners enjoy this new sort of stroke.

A student once said that when she started rubbing her man with a slow and light stroke, his penis lost its erection. There are a number of factors that could be involved here, but, basically, she has to take responsibility for the loss of engorgement. First, she does not even have to touch it to make it erect. She might have doubted how much pleasure she could give him, remembering some past experience in which she tried but failed to give him pleasure or an orgasm. Doubt, like anger, nullifies turn-on: When her attention is on her doubt, guess where her attention is not? —that's right, on her partner. Second, she could have enjoyed touching a flaccid penis and gotten into agreement that she did not want to have an engorged penis on her hands at that moment.

She does best when she can put her attention on the pleasure and turn-on that she does feel. She can become playful and tease him, saying she will barely touch him and will make him quiver and quake at her will. She can touch him only when it brings pleasure to her hand, and she can let him know how wonderful his penis feels. She can let him know that she will squirt him on her own terms, that while his penis is hard in her hands, it belongs to her. Take ownership and control, and keep the communication lines open. This enables him to relax, as he does not have to wonder about what you're doing or what you're up to. Frequent communication also allows you to stay in present time and not go into doubt. Only "do him" for as long as it is pleasurable. The goal is not ejaculation but pleasure with each stroke. A woman may want to give a man pleasure, but she has to do it in a way that makes it fun, not a chore or a duty.

When he experiences great pleasure, you will have to peak him to keep him from ejaculating. If you are new to doing a man, you can ask him to let you know when he is about to ejaculate. You may also observe a secondary erection (see FIGURE 5.2, earlier in the book). The head of the penis becomes more engorged and bulbous. It may turn a dark

purple. You can also smell the semen as he gets close to squirting. Through experience, you will learn how far you can take him without bringing him to ejaculation. You will learn how best to peak him at the different points preceding ejaculation. If he has not gone into the expulsion phase of the ejaculatory response, you can peak him by stopping or changing the stroke. If he has started to squirt or is right on the verge, you can bring him back down by pressing on the ejaculatory-duct area, right under his scrotum (see FIGURE 5.3, earlier). The farther he has gone into the ejaculation phase, the more pressure that is required. There is a point when even using a lot of pressure fails to stop the ejaculation. In fact, pressing after a certain point may actually keep the ejaculation from being as pleasurable as it could have been, making it end in a small instead of a big bang. If this happens, it is somewhat unfortunate, but remember that you are learning how far you can take him, and if you have to waste or lessen some of his ejaculations in order to become finely attuned in the future, it is worth some spilled semen.

It is best to be in control when your partner ejaculates instead of letting his ejaculation take you by surprise. The more often you do your man, the better you'll be at realizing when to stop and peak him and when to start again. At some point, you may decide to take him over the edge and let him ejaculate. Bring him as high as you want, and then take him through the ejaculation. Keep giving him strokes as he ejaculates. Some men like lighter pressure and a slower stroke as they squirt. You can actually prolong his pleasure by gradually lightening and slowing the stroke during the ejaculation. (Review the section "Approaching Ejaculation" in the chapter "Receiving an EMO" for more pointers about this stage of his experience.) Keep feeling the sensations in your hand, and as long as it feels good to you, continue to stroke. Don't forget to continue the communication while he squirts. Let him know how much you like it and how it feels.

✐ Coming Together ✐

In the "Positions" chapter, we described a few of our favorite positions for coming together. In fact, you can use any position that you like in which both partners' genitals are accessible to each other at the same time. However, before you try coming together, it is imperative that both you and your partner learn how to do each other one at a time. When two people simultaneously focus their attention on one person's orgasm, it enhances the environment for deliberate training and optimizes the orgasm. You also must become familiar with your partner's genital anatomy, preferences, and idiosyncrasies before attempting to come together. (You can do this with some of the exercises described in the "Pressures" chapter, later in the book.)

Once you have mastered both the doing and the getting done and have become friends with your partner's genitals, you are ready to conquer the demons and monsters of coming together. Competition for attention, selfishness, and feelings of unworthiness are what causes the "coming-together demons" to thrive. If you think that your partner should put more attention on your genitals, or if you wonder whether to feel your genitals or to put more attention on the genitals of your partner, you are in your head, rather than feeling. This is when the "monsters" get you. Now is the time to communicate, and even to take a break if appropriate. You want to be able both to receive and to give attention graciously, without feeling or thinking that you are in need of attention or are unworthy of it. Whenever you feel needy or unworthy, the demons trap you. You can tame or disarm them if you remain enthusiastic, enjoy yourself with every stroke, do what feels best, and communicate thoroughly.

Communication is of the utmost importance in any sexual activity, and it is even more essential when coming together. If there is a gap in your communication, even for a short time, you leave a space through which the demons can enter the picture. By the same token, you can exorcise these demons with proper and precise communication. When done right, coming together can be one of the most gratifying sexual experiences you can have.

Coming together is especially helpful to women who are interested in learning about the most pleasurable and fun ways to interact with a man's genitals. The most enjoyable way to deal with anything, including genitals, is via orgasm. These sexual activities give a woman the opportunity to do just that.

Before you start this exercise it is a good idea to agree on how long you will be doing it. Once you reach the time limit, you can always go longer if you both agree. Once the two of you are in position, use the same techniques for doing each other together that you would when doing each other one at a time. For the best results, the man starts doing the woman first; only after she is coming easily does she begin to do him. Why does the woman's pleasure start first? There are several reasons. First, it helps the man feel productive and "gentlemanly" if he first stimulates the woman, and it helps the woman relate pleasurably to the man's genitals if she's already in orgasm. Then, when she starts doing him, the man feels even better because his pleasure is being focused upon as well. First he teases her, lubricates her, and plays with her genitals just as he would in a regular do. Once she is fully orgasmic, she can take his penis in her hand and begin lubricating him as he continues to do her.

When you do this technique properly, energy circulates through your two bodies in a way that is analogous to energy in a cyclotron. The more you appreciate and acknowledge what is happening in your body and in your partner's body, the higher you both can go.

MONSTERING ⇨ A man and a woman agree to have a date to come together using the "two-headed monster" position. They are both right-handed, so they both lie on their left sides with their heads facing in opposite directions. They agree that the man will start to do the woman first, and that when she is getting off well, she will start to do him. They gather the pillows they need. The man chooses two large pillows to support his back. He picks a medium-size pillow to place on the woman's thigh and a small pillow to place on top of her abdomen, where he will rest his doing arm. The woman places a pillow under her outside thigh. She also gets a large pillow that she can position to support her back when she moves from lying on her back to lying on her side. She chooses a medium-size pillow to put over the man's inner thigh, which will support her when she rests her torso there, and a small pillow to place under her head. They place their drinks nearby as well as two jars of their favorite lubricant, Albolene (one jar for each of them), and a couple of towels. They agree to stay in this position for twenty-five minutes, and they set the alarm clock accordingly.

They start with the woman lying on her back and the man lying on his left side, with the two large pillows stuffed behind his back. He places his left hand under the woman's buttocks, resting his forearm between her legs. He rests his torso on a pillow placed over her left thigh. His right hand is free to reach for the Albolene, and he can rest his right forearm on the small pillow on her abdomen.

He begins by sensually touching her thighs, moving his right hand close to her pubic area and then retreating. He teases her pubic hair with his wrist and with the back and front of his hand (see FIGURES 2.2 AND 2.3, earlier in the book). He plays with her inner labia using light, teasing touches. He lets her know that he is going to put some lubricant on her. He spreads the lubricant, starting on the perineum and working his way toward the clitoris via the inner labia. Just below the clitoris, he pauses and retreats; he does this a few times. He removes his hand to get a little more lubricant on his index finger and then puts it directly on her favorite spot on her clitoris.

He anchors her hood with his right thumb and easily hooks his right index finger on the slick upper left quadrant of the head of her clitoris. He starts to take her up with a light, short, fairly quick and steady stroke. The woman really enjoys his attention and his touch and acknowledges all the marvelous sensations that she experiences. He lets her know that her clitoris is getting redder, engorged, and harder. He tells her how wonderful she feels and smells. He peaks her by using a slightly slower stroke and then takes her up with this new stroke. He takes her for a couple more peaks. She is now in full orgasm.

She tells him that she is now going to put her hands on his cock. She rolls over to her left side and stuffs the big pillow behind her. He continues to stroke her and reminds her to feel her clitoris. She puts a pillow over his inner thigh and rests the left side of her torso on it. She gets some lubricant from her jar and delicately rubs some over his entire penis. She lets him know that his penis is hard and hot. He lets her know how wonderful her hands feel on it. She tells him that she will hold his penis in her hand and squeeze it gently. She lets him know how wonderful it feels in her hand and also how good her clitoris feels.

She circles his cock with her hand and starts stroking up and down, quite slowly and deliberately, giving him long strokes. She lightens her touch as she goes over his apex and corona. They are both getting higher together, talking continuously about how fantastic they feel. They stop at the same time for a peak and a sip of water. They relate how much fun they are both having and put their heads back in each other's crotch for another climbing peak. They keep going higher. Each feels that they are like one body getting off together. They peak each other a few more times, each time stopping and starting together.

The man is lying on his back now, more relaxed but still stroking her clitoris with his finger. Her orgasm is taking him higher, and his is taking her higher at the same time. She tells him that she is going to make him ejaculate on the next peak and there is nothing he can do to stop her. She takes him higher and higher even as he continues to take her higher. She lets him know how good he has made her pussy feel. He gets a secondary erection, the head of his penis bulging out and turning red and purple. She continues to stroke as he begins to squirt in her hands. She lightens her touch but continues to stroke him, ever more slowly, to extend his orgasm as long as it will last. They lie in sheer ecstasy for a while; then he rolls back onto his side and gives her a pull-up (described in Chapter 10) as she continues to have strong contractions. They towel each other off just as the alarm rings.

We have presented quite a bit of information on how to receive and give an orgasm. We have still more information and techniques to offer, though, and the next three chapters describe how to use pressures, how to incorporate your second hand into your pleasure, and how best to bring your partner down after taking them on this orgasmic ride.

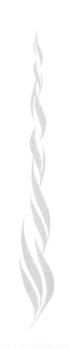

CHAPTER EIGHT

In our classes, we teach that pleasure and pain result from each individual's interpretation of certain pressures. Once, I visited our dentist just after he had taken our class, and as he was drilling a big hole in my tooth, he casually recited that pain and pleasure were just my interpretation of pressure. I laughed through the pain.

Pressures

We don't suggest that every sensation can be made to feel pleasurable. Our bodies contain specific pain receptors that when stimulated evoke pain. These are called *nociceptors*. Our bodies also contain, however, touch-sensitive and pressure-sensitive nerve receptors that can sometimes feel pleasure and other times feel discomfort. When these are stimulated, some people really enjoy the sensation, but others shriek with pain. The difference is influenced by how much acceptance and resistance are demonstrated by the person who is touched; by personal history and the associations the person has with different touches and pressures; and by how much trust the person places in the one who touches him and whether he believes that the person knows what she is doing.

To our knowledge, there are no specific pleasure receptors, no receptors that interpret every stimulus as wonderful. Our brains, however, can be considered the ultimate pleasure receptors. The pleasure mechanism in the brain is driven by the activity of different hormones—for example, the endorphins that are usually released when the body engages in familiar activities such as sex, eating, or exercise. Many drugs, such as opiates, imitate these natural hormones; this may be the reason for these substances' highly addictive quality.

If a person has negative associations about past sexual experiences, they may encounter difficulty with present-day sexual activities. Some people can decide to change their own minds so that they become able to enjoy new sensual relationships, but others may be so stuck that they must undergo years of therapy before they can start interpreting sensual touch as pleasurable.

Crises result from a resistance to change, and resistance to touch is felt as pain. When you are touched, you experience a change in sensation, and although it may not qualify as a crisis, the more resistance you feel, the more negative your experience of touch will be. But by being relaxed and anticipating every sensation, you can pleasurably experience a wide range of pressures, from a gentle breeze to a sharp slap. The genitals, specifically the clitoris and the penis, have the highest concentration of nerve endings on our bodies; thus, they are the most receptive to experiencing a wide range of touch sensations.

EXERCISE 1: Touching for Pleasure

To experience an EMO, your mind must find as much pleasure as possible in every stroke. You have the ability to turn different parts of your body on or off at will. Here is a little exercise in turning on different body parts one at a time, which you can practice with your partner.

Sit on the floor or on a bed, facing each other. One person will be the "toucher" and the other the "touchee," and then you can switch positions. The toucher asks if he or she can touch a specific body part. It can be anything from your left eyebrow to the back of your right hand to your penis or clitoris. You may want to agree to leave out the genitals at first, to avoid feeling any pressure. (You can even do this exercise with your clothes on, but it probably will be more fun with them off.) You, the touchee, can say yes or no. The toucher thanks you in either case. They then proceed to touch you only if your answer was yes. If the toucher wishes to touch your back, or a leg that is out of reach, and you answer yes, make it easy for the toucher by offering your back or uncrossing your leg, or doing whatever is necessary to accommodate the request.

The toucher touches with one hand, feeling as much pleasure as he or she can without stroking, just touching or holding the body part for a few seconds. The toucher then withdraws the hand and again thanks you. You, the touchee, take the opportunity to "turn on" the body part in question — that is, to feel as much as you can from the touch. By putting a lot of attention there and anticipating pleasure, you will feel the most from each touch. You can test this by deliberately *not* putting your attention on feeling the pleasure, and then focusing attention on the touch once again. This allows you to see how much responsibility you have for making a touch feel great, or not feel so great. Continue for five minutes or so, and then switch positions.

In our classes, we instruct the touchee to intentionally say no to some of the requests. This way, the toucher gets to experience resistance and can ask to touch the same part again. A variation on this exercise is for the touchee to ask the toucher to touch a specific body part. This time the toucher can say yes or no. Make sure you turn on the body part that you want touched. These exercises help you to learn to ask for what you want and to overcome resistance, as well as to turn on a specific part of your body.

EXERCISE 2: Pressure Testing

Another exercise we teach offers a good way for students to investigate different pressures of touch and to take pleasure from many different pressures. The goal of the exercise is to find the range of pressures, from light to heavy, that feels good on a particular body part. You are not looking for the one best pressure, although if your partner tells you that one feels best, that is an added bonus.

The first few times that our students do this exercise, we instruct them not to touch each other's genitals but to select another area of the body, one that carries less "charge" than the private parts do. This area can be the hand, the arm, the leg, the foot, or whatever both partners agree upon before beginning. Once you and your partner pick a body part, stick with it and define the area you will touch. We will use the left foot as an example.

After getting your partner's agreement, let your partner know that you are going to touch the bottom arch of his or her left foot with your thumb (or another finger). Use a light pressure; then ask if your partner would like more pressure. If the answer is yes, increase the pressure by a small increment. Repeat the question, and increase the pressure each time your partner says yes. There will come a point at which your partner does not want to receive any more pressure or when you don't feel like giving any more.

Let your partner know that you are going to move to a different spot on the left foot. Pick another part of the foot—let's say the top of the foot between the big toe and the second toe—and start pressing there, telling your partner what you will do before you do it. Pressure test as many body parts and areas as you and your partner agree to test. You could put your hand around a finger or a toe and squeeze progressively tighter. You could pull on a finger, an earlobe, or any other part you've agreed to test.

Once you have the knack of doing this and you are adept at the necessary communication techniques, you can move on to the genitals, pressure testing all the areas of your partner's private anatomy. See the next exercise for tips on how to do this.

EXERCISE 3: Genital Pressure Testing

When pressure testing a woman's genitals, you can start wherever you like. Let's use the inner labia as an example. As you did with the foot, once you have agreed upon an area, inform your partner that you will press her inner left labia between your thumb and forefinger. Start with a light squeeze and ask whether you should increase the pressure; continue until either you or she does not want to go farther. See how far you can pull the labia out from the body, remembering to proceed in small increments. Then move to the other labia.

You can put a finger on her perineum and see how much pressure she can pleasurably take there. You can pull on her pubic hair. You can squeeze the hood of the clitoris between thumb and finger and experiment with increasing pressures. You can even check out the clitoris itself. Squeeze the accessible portion of the clitoral shaft, or even slap the clitoris if she enjoys that. With your partner's agreement, pressure test whatever areas you like. You will be amazed by how much pressure some of these areas can receive and still feel good. Avoid reaching any kind of pain.

This is a wonderful way to explore her genitals, and you can be as creative or curious as you want to be. Most women love this kind of attention; you may even notice contractions, engorgement, and other signs of orgasm.

When it comes to testing different pressures on a man's genitals, do anything you like as long as you get his agreement first. You can pull on his testicles to see how much pleasurable pull he can take. Some guys are macho, and so remember that you are not looking for the most he can take—just the most *pleasurable* amount. You can squeeze his penis, progressing in small increments. You can stretch out the scrotal sac in opposite directions. You can tug on his pubic hair. As long as you get his agreement, start lightly, and progress slowly, all these will be pleasurable experiments.

It is also fun to explore your partner's pressure limitations at the other extreme, on the delicate side. Experiment with the lightest of touches to see if your partner can feel them. You can play with a feather, tickling both her erogenous zones and his. Or try the stroke that Dr. Vic Baranco calls the "black lace." Put a glob of lubricant on your fingertip; it needs to be a rather viscous kind of lubricant, rather than a thin, runny sort. Without putting your finger directly on the clitoris, instead touch the lubricant to the clitoris (FIGURE 8.1). It's important to use enough lubricant; use a glob that's big enough that a light positioned behind it shines through it.

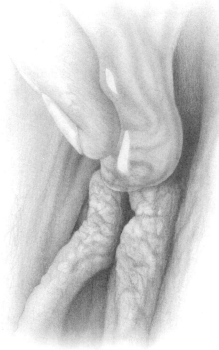

FIGURE 8.1
Creating indirect contact with the clitoris by touching finger on a glob of lubricant that was placed on the clitoris

Note that your finger is positioned on one side of the lubricant and her clitoris is on the opposite side. When you move your finger, the lubricant also moves, indirectly stimulating the clitoris. This is a great stroke to use on a woman who thinks she is supersensitive and that direct contact on her clitoris is too much. She feels a slight pressure from the lubricant and eventually may feel safe enough to allow increasing amounts of direct pressure. You can also check out the black-lace stroke on the apex of the penis. Again, put a glob of lubricant on your finger and touch his most sensitive area with only the lubricant. Most men are not super-sensitive, so experiment to see how little pressure he is able to feel.

When you're doing a woman, one way to extend a nice peak is to use a gradually lighter and slower stroke. This allows her to take the peak even higher than it was before. This is a technique to use occasionally, rather than on every peak.

EXERCISE 4: Investigating for Smell, Taste, and Sight

Besides touching your partner's genitals, you can use your senses of sight, smell, and taste to get to know them better. Make sure to first get your partner's agreement and to use lots of communication when using any of these methods. It works best when the person who's being investigated is relaxed and tells the investigator how he or she feels at each step. The "touchee" can report all pleasurable sensations, including which ones feel best. The touchee must communicate especially well when he or she is orally investigated.

The investigator can lick for taste and also apply sucking pressure to find out where a partner likes to be sucked, and with how much pressure. The investigator describes what they will do before they do it. Then, after each step, the investigator reports how the experience feels and what they see, smell, and taste. If your partner plans to smell and taste your genital and anal areas, it is probably a good idea to first take a shower, unless you know your partner's olfactory limits to be expansive and inclusive. This goes for both men and women.

When exploring the male genitalia, you can put your mouth on his scrotum or penis to taste and to test how much sucking pressure feels good to him. He has to do most of the communicating in this position, as your mouth is occupied. You can do whatever you please to him as long as you have his agreement. The more things you can think up to do and test, the better acquainted you will become with his private parts.

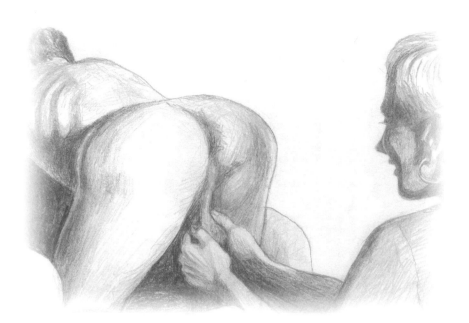

FIGURE 8.2
**Investigating
his genitals
from the rear**

You can examine your partner from both the back and the front. To investigate a woman's front side, have her sit on a couch and spread her legs apart as you kneel on a pillow in front of her. To research the back side of your partner's genitals, have her kneel on a couch or a large chair, facing the back of the couch and arching her back, while you kneel on the floor on a pillow. Make sure you have appropriate lighting so you can investigate thoroughly. Examine your partner with curiosity and enthusiasm. Do whatever investigation you can dream up, as long as you communicate and your partner agrees to it.

This couch position is also good for investigating a man's rear view (FIGURE 8.2). You can investigate his front side by kneeling on a pillow before him while he stands up. You can look at, smell, taste, and touch him from both sides.

Now that we have given you ways to determine the appropriate pressure to use in any circumstance, it is time to see what you can do with your second hand. The second, or "nondoing" hand, is the one that usually does not directly stroke the clitoris or penis, and so it is free to try other techniques (including varying levels of pressure) on secondary areas, all of which can make the EMO feel even better.

CHAPTER NINE

The word vagina means "sheath" or "purse," a place or space in which to put something. It is a male-oriented definition; from this perspective, the something that is meant to fill a vagina is a penis. That is what "sex" is about—the insertion of a penis into a vagina, a form into a hole—and the goal is reproduction. In its many varieties, sex has been nature's way of continuing the species. It obviously must be pleasurable, since it has worked so well in so many animals. But the fact remains that many women don't have orgasms during intercourse: the vaginal wall itself lacks nerve endings that feel pressure. However, there are nerves in the underlying tissue that can feel pleasurable stimulation. This chapter describes and illustrates how to stimulate these areas with the hands.

Insertion, or What to Do with the Second Hand

Orgasm During Intercourse?

When a penis penetrates a vagina, what happens is a total surrounding of the male's organ by soft, smooth, and delightfully pulsating flesh. It is like a sheath to his sword, a purse to his coins (or loins). The nerve endings of his member are stimulated in 360 degrees. He can be driven to orgasm in a matter of seconds.

This is great, if the goal is reproduction and the woman wants his semen. The problem is that although the penis and all its nerve endings are stimulated, the vaginal wall itself has no nerve receptors for pressure, only temperature receptors for heat and cold. This is why most women do not have orgasms during intercourse. As a choice for recreational or nonreproductive sex, intercourse is far from the best way for women to reach orgasm.

Some women, however, are able to reach orgasm through penetration with a penis. This usually requires that the clitoris is somehow stimulated by the motion of the penis and the vagina. A couple of factors can affect this. On some women, the distance between the clitoris and the introitus is very short. The closer the clitoris lies to the vaginal opening, the more likely that it is stimulated by a penis going in and out. Also, if a woman is properly stimulated by hand or mouth before insertion, the engorgement of the vulva area causes the clitoris to move toward the introitus. Or the movement of the penis can also engage the labia, which are connected to the hood of the clitoris in some women. This labial movement causes the hood to move up and down against the clitoris, possibly resulting in an orgasm, almost as if she were having intercourse with herself.

Another possibility is that a woman has built a connection between her inner lips or introital area and her clitoris, using the connections exercise that was given in the "Masturbation" chapter, earlier in the book. Then, when her labia and introitus are stimulated with the penis, she also experiences the sensation in her clitoris, allowing her to reach orgasm.

Some women report success with a method that involves positioning themselves so that their clitoris lies against the man's pubic symphysis, which is covered by his pubic mons, which is itself cushioned with a layer of fat.

Her clitoris is now positioned between her symphysis and his. This is called *clitoral seizure*. At the end of each inward stroke of his penis, whether he is moving or she is moving, she gives a little downward and outward rotation of her pelvis, which presses her clitoris firmly between the bones and then rubs it upward. This is called *clitoral excursion*. Together, clitoral seizure and excursion move the clitoris downward as the penis inserts itself inward, and moves it upward as the penis pulls outward. The clitoral glans rubs along the man's padded pubic bone, and the clitoral shaft is given a downward and then an upward tug. The clitoris moves only about an inch, depending on clitoral size, shape, and the woman's skill at this maneuver. A woman can do this movement in any position, but she has most freedom of movement if she's on top or on her side.

The penis, although highly sensitive, is not known for its dexterity; still, a woman can position herself during intercourse to stimulate those nerves that can register pleasure. Such positions usually involve the woman being on top or at the man's side, depending on her acrobatic abilities. If she wishes to stimulate the G-spot, having the man enter her from behind while she is on her knees can be effective. We offer more details about the G-spot a little later in the chapter.

Placement of the Second Hand on a Woman Doee

Because the clitoris has by far the most nerve endings and is the seat of all orgasm for women, it is in her interest to have her clitoris directly stimulated whenever she desires intense pleasure. She can either stroke her own clitoris with her hand during intercourse or have her partner stroke it. The dexterous hands are much better equipped than the penis to stimulate not only the clitoris but also the nerve endings deep inside the vagina that can add to a woman's orgasm. (The word *dexterous* means "manually skillful" or "adroit." It actually means "right-handed" in Latin, but that was their prejudice.) The best way for the doer to stimulate these inner vaginal areas on a female doee

FIGURE 9.1
Separation of fingers in a V to allow placement of two fingers under each buttock cheek

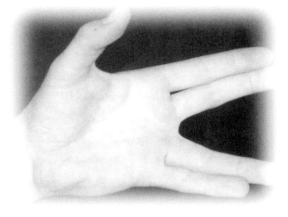

FIGURE 9.2
Thumb of second hand resting snugly at the base of a woman's introitus

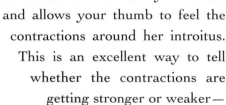

is with the "non-doing," or bottom, hand while continuing to stroke her clitoris with the primary, or "doing," hand. Remember that doing involves two hands; the second hand has a number of roles and purposes.

We like to begin doing most women with the second, non-clitoral-stimulating hand in a specific position. Place your hand palm-up under the woman's buttocks and spread your fingers in a V, with two fingers on each of her derriere cheeks (FIGURE 9.1). Get your hand as far as necessary under her buttocks to allow the space between forefinger and thumb to rest snugly against her perineum. Now snugly place your thumb at the base or bottom of her introitus, pad down, but without penetrating the vagina (FIGURE 9.2). In this position you have a good, firm grip on her bottom. This allows the woman to relax into your hands and allows your thumb to feel the contractions around her introitus. This is an excellent way to tell whether the contractions are getting stronger or weaker— that is, whether she is going up or down. You are also in an excellent position to tell whether and how much she tenses up or relaxes.

THE G-SPOT ⇔ Everyone is always asking us about the G-spot. The term *G-spot* was coined in 1950 by Dr. Ernest Gräfenburg to refer to the spongy area at the front of the vaginal wall. Again, the vaginal wall lacks specific nerve receptors, but the nerves that innervate the clitoris run into the clitoral root, which attaches near the end of the vaginal canal, on the front of the vaginal wall. We call this area of the vagina "twelve o'clock." This area can be stimulated with one or two fingers in a number of ways.

To use two fingers, separate them slightly to avoid stroking the exact center or twelve o'clock area; position the hand palm up, with the fingers penetrating the vagina fairly deeply, to a depth of about two inches, or two-thirds the length of your fingers (FIGURE 9.3). Now stroke or massage the spongy, bulbous tissue that you can feel on the roof (if the woman is lying on her back) or at the front of the vagina. Move your fingers in almost a come-hither motion. Avoid stroking the precise center of the G-spot, because the urethral canal runs in this vicinity, and stimulating it can cause some women to feel the need to urinate. On the other hand, some women may actually enjoy having this area stroked, so check with your partner.

You can also use one finger to stroke one side of the twelve o'clock area at a time. Another technique is to place one or two fingers with your palm pointing downward, toward the back wall of the vagina (what we call "six o'clock"); and use the backs of your fingers to stimulate the vaginal roof, or G-spot, area.

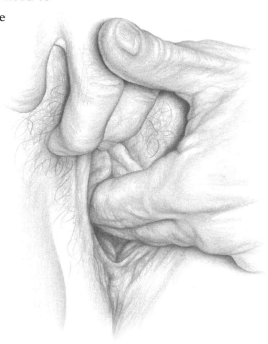

FIGURE 9.3
Two fingers of left hand inserted, just left and right of twelve o'clock

OTHER SPOTS The six o'clock area, mentioned above, is another spot in the vagina that deserves and enjoys attention. Position the non-doing hand as described at the beginning of this section, with the thumb resting at the base or bottom of the doee's introitus. Make sure her introitus is lubricated. While the doing hand plays with the clitoris, the thumb can rest on the introitus or it can play with the inner lips, introitus, and perineum. The thumb can apply pressure to the introitus or stroke it lightly, depending on what the woman likes and what feels best.

If your partner "invites" your thumb inside her vagina (she may do this either verbally or by "drawing in" the thumb with her vagina), the thumb will be in the six o'clock position (FIGURE 9.4). You can massage that area

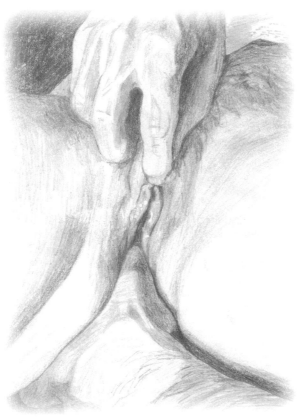

FIGURE 9.4
Thumb "invited in" at six o'clock position

with your thumb or just rest the thumb inside the vagina. You can use various pressures, from light to firm, to stimulate the nerves from her anal area that course through the vaginal walls at the six o'clock area. You can rub the roof of the vagina or the G-spot area with the back of your thumb. If you turn your non-doing hand over, you can press down with the pads of one, two, or more fingers to stimulate the six o'clock area (FIGURE 9.5). You can use a variety of pressures or move the fingers in an in-and-out stroke. You can even press down firmly with your fingers, teasing your partner by telling her that you are going to "pin her to the bed."

You can run two or more fingers along the floor of the vagina, as far as they will go, still at the six o'clock position. Move the fingers in and out along the vaginal floor, either slowly or quickly, feeling the pleasure of each movement. This action stimulates more nerves, which are embedded near the spinal cord. However, do this only if the woman is fully receptive, so that her vagina is fully stretched by adequate sensual stimulation. Make sure that you press downward rather than backward, as you do not want to bang against the cervix, which is located at the far end of the vagina.

The vagina houses two deep pockets on its left and right sides, located around three o'clock and nine o'clock, respectively. Right-handed doers can easily reach the three o'clock side by placing the index and middle fingers of the left hand against the left wall of the vagina. There you will feel the pocket; stroke it with an in-and-out or a come-hither movement (FIGURE 9.6). Left-handed doers have easier access to the nine o'clock side with their right hand. You can also use the thumb to reach the pocket on the side that is more difficult for you to reach with your fingers (FIGURE 9.7). These pockets may be located closer to three-thirty or four o'clock, and eight-thirty and eight o'clock, in some women; go wherever you feel the deepest pocket and wherever it feels best to place your fingers.

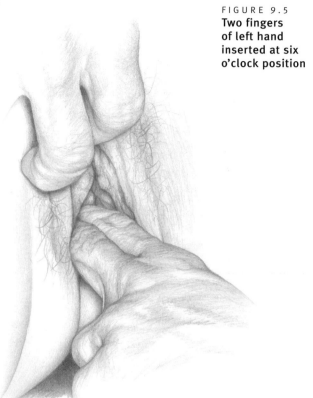

FIGURE 9.5
Two fingers of left hand inserted at six o'clock position

FIGURE 9.6
**Two fingers
of left hand
inserted at
three o'clock
position**

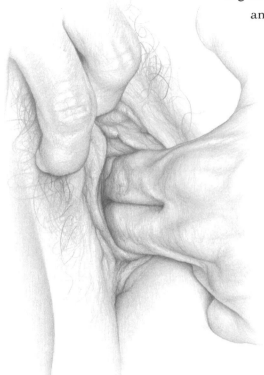

One of my favorite strokes involves inserting two fingers, pads up, against the G-spot, and then using the thumb of my inserting (or non-doing) hand to pull back on the clitoral hood. This way, I surround the clitoris from four sides: from underneath, from above, from the side with the anchoring thumb (you can also remove the anchoring thumb and let the other thumb do all the retracting), and with the finger directly on the clitoral head.

Once a person is stimulated to a high intensity, he or she might enjoy having the lower abdomen and pubic area, or mons pubis, massaged with pressure at the same time that you continue stimulating either the penis or the clitoris. On a woman, massage the area between her clitoris and a few inches below her navel, moving up and down with firm pressure. Some men also like to have this area stimulated when they are at a high peak.

There is also the option of inserting your whole hand inside the vagina. This is something we do not practice or teach, but a blind man who attended one of our groups described how he did it. He said that he first inserted one finger, then a second, then a third, and then the pinky. When the woman opened and relaxed even more, he tucked his thumb under his hand and inserted that, too. Now he had his whole hand or fist inside her, and it all felt good to him and to her. This is for a woman who likes heavy pressure; she must be in agreement with it before you proceed. It is known as "fist fucking" in slang.

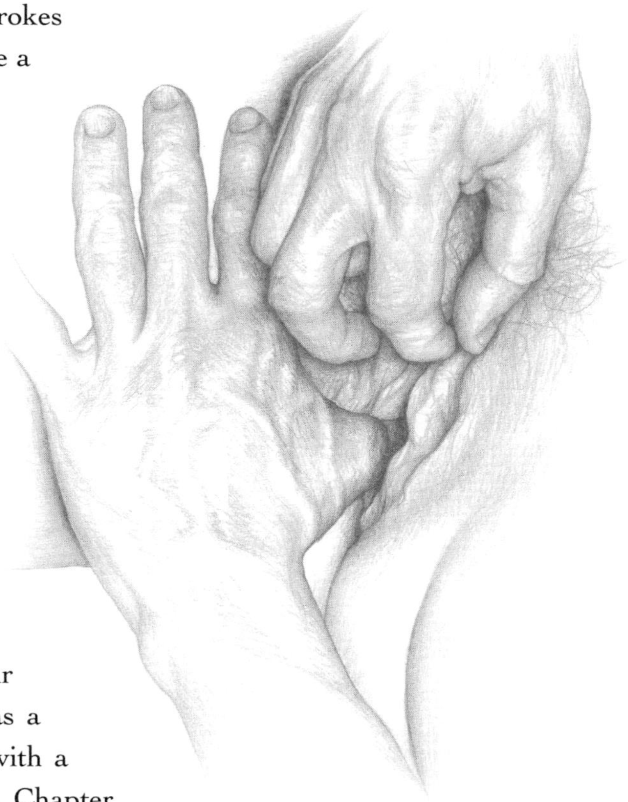

With any of the insertion strokes we have described, you can use a variety of speeds, pressures, or motions. You can leave your finger or thumb in an area and barely move it, or you can massage the area with a quick in-and-out stroke. You can use either light pressure or a lot of pressure. You can move the fingers all the way, or a just a little bit, in and out. You can stroke in circles or with a come-hither motion. You can use insertion as an adjunct to help you take your partner higher on a peak or as a tool to bring them down, as with a pull-up (which is described in Chapter 10). Do whatever feels best to you and your partner. Explore the different possibilities with enthusi-

FIGURE 9.7
Thumb of left hand inserted at nine o'clock position

asm and inquisitiveness. There is no formula that works every time. Sometimes your partner wants lots of pressure, and other times she might not want any insertion at all. By keeping your attention on your partner, you are able to feel what to do and to remain in full control of the orgasm. Remember that the majority of a woman's sensation comes from the clitoris; consequently, we almost always continue to stroke her there even as we use the insertion strokes. The pressure used on the clitoris or even the penis for that matter will usually be less than the pressure being used on areas stimulated with one's second hand.

We are not suggesting that people stop having intercourse. There is something very erotic and intimate about it. Intercourse is usually done hard and fast, but the slower you do it, the more you can actually feel. And there are ways, such as those discussed at the beginning of this chapter, for a woman to position herself and to move that allow her to feel more during intercourse; it especially helps if she is engorged and orgasmic before penetration. Intercourse is also a very effective means of coming down. Both partners can give and receive a great deal of pressure during intercourse; this is a great way to detumesce. Read more about this in Chapter 10.

Placement of the Second Hand on a Man Doee

Numerous opportunities exist for your second hand when you're stroking a man's penis with your primary one. If the man is uncircumcised, you can use the second hand to pull down the foreskin. Form a ring or semi-ring with your index or middle finger and thumb. Circle the penis, and bring the ring as far as you can toward the base of the penis. Hold the bottom of the penis with this ring as you stroke with your primary hand. (This also feels good to a circumcised man; see FIGURE 4.22, earlier in the book.) You can press down firmly with the second hand, and even use its free fingers to play with his scrotum.

You can also use your second hand directly on his penis in concert with the primary hand; these techniques are outlined in the "Doing a Man" section of the "Giving an EMO" chapter.

THE SCROTUM AND SURROUNDING AREAS Most men enjoy having you play with their scrotum while you stroke them on the penis. (This is where the information you've gathered from the exercise in the preceding chapter on genital pressure testing comes in handy. Many men like having the scrotum pulled away from the body with varying amounts of pressure (see FIGURE 7.7, earlier in the book). Don't pull directly on the testes, but rather on the scrotal skin behind or in front of the testes. Also try stroking the scrotal sac. Most things you can imagine and try out will feel great as long as you avoid pushing the scrotum and testes into the body with a lot of pressure.

Men also find it very pleasurable to have the area behind the scrotum rubbed. Externally, this is where the perineum is located; internally, the area houses the "hidden cock," the prostate, and the ejaculatory duct. When the penis is erect, you can feel the engorged hidden cock. Many men like quite a bit of pressure here. You can stroke this area with your second hand in concert with stroking the penis. You can feel the hidden cock with your fingers and stroke it in sync with the primary hand's movements on the visible penis. You can press into the area with your fingers or even knuckles and play with different pressures (see FIGURE 2.1, earlier in the book). Some men like a partner to press this area with a knee or even the heel of the foot, so obviously it can take a lot of pressure. This is the same area that, when pressed hard, can stop a man from squirting. The difference between taking him higher and peaking him lies in the specific intention you manifest through your strokes. You can continue to stroke the hidden cock or to exert pressure on the perineum as he ejaculates; when doing so, you should really be able to feel the strength of his contractions.

CONNECTIONS ⌇ You can use the second hand to build connections between the penis (or the clitoris) and any other part of the body. Use the techniques presented in the "Connections" exercise in the "Masturbation" chapter, only now do them to your partner rather than to yourself. Essentially, you use your second hand to stroke another part of your partner's body while you simultaneously stroke the penis or clitoris. The secondary area can be another part of the genitals—such as the scrotum, perineum, or introitus—or any other reachable part, such as a thigh or nipple. Now alternately remove your hand from either the primary or the secondary area.

Both partners need to employ appropriate communications throughout this procedure. Whenever the doee stops feeling sensation, he or she must communicate that fact to the doer, and the doee must also tell the doer when to start stroking the primary or secondary area once again. The more you practice this technique—either alone or with a partner—the more your ability to feel a connection will increase.

ANAL STIMULATION ❧ Many gay men use the anus as an orifice in intercourse. The anus and the anal area house the body's second-highest concentration of nerve endings, so during anal intercourse both men can simultaneously experience pleasure. In order to experience the best EMO, however, the hands are still the best choice. Your partner's anus can be stimulated at the same time you are playing with his penis; this is a great way to stimulate these two highly sensitive areas at once.

When playing with someone's anus, it is best to proceed slowly. Trim your fingernails beforehand. Some people clean out their anus with an enema if they know in advance that they will be anally stimulated. Many men and women are sensitive and squeamish about having their anuses penetrated. Only enter an orifice if it is receptive and inviting. Never poke to get in; doing so can cause pain and abrasion. Because of the high concentration of nerve endings, it can feel really wonderful to have the outside of the anus played with and stimulated. Use a little lubricant on the tip of your finger and make circular strokes around the anus in a sensual manner while at the same time stimulating the penis or clitoris with your other hand. Stroke however feels best to your hand, whether you're moving up and down, side to side, or circularly. After the doee has been pleasurably touched for a time on the outside of the anus and is getting off well, the doee is more likely to open up and desire penetration. On a man, you can now stroke the prostate area from inside the anus. Ensure your finger is lubricated, then insert it (pad up) fairly deeply and massage in a come-hither motion. The goal is not insertion or getting deeply inside, but rather to make it feel good and pleasurable.

When playing with a woman's anus, do not use the same finger inside her vagina that you used in her anus; this is important so as to prevent the spread of bacterial or other types of infections. I usually use my pinky or ring finger to stimulate the anus and save my other two fingers and thumb for inside the vagina (FIGURE 9.8).

Although most peo-
ple know the differ-
ence between their
orifices, the anus
has been mistaken
as the vagina by
more than one
couple. We knew
a couple who tried
for more than five years
to have a baby. Then
they took a sensuality
course and learned a few
things. They found out that
they had been doing it in the wrong orifice the whole time.
(They were both college graduates.) They consequently found the vagina
and had children.

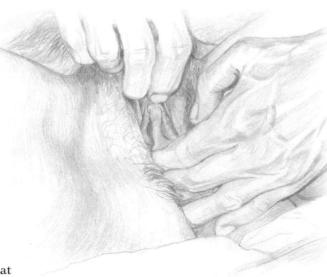

FIGURE 9.8
**Ring finger
inserted into
anus**

*The pleasure available from stimulation of other body parts during stimu-
lation of the primary zones is a topic most people are uninformed about.
Including some of the practices we have presented here in their sensual life
is a way for a couple to create more pleasure for themselves. Skilled use of
the second hand not only increases the fun and pleasure in a sensual experience but is an important tool in helping the doer to gauge the level of
tumescence and determine where the orgasm is headed at each moment. Once
you've determined this, it is good to be prepared with some methods for taking your partner down. The next chapter describes how and when to do this.*

CHAPTER TEN

Down is just a direction, yet the word has many negative connotations. Hell is located down below us. When someone feels sad, he is down. Putting someone down means saying bad things about her. We could continue pointing out examples, but we don't want to bring you too far down.

Coming Down

To come down during an orgasm is not a bad situation. Everything about orgasm can be wonderful. Every time you peak someone, you are deliberately bringing them down. This means that in any one orgasm, many downs can occur, as well as many ups. Some sexologists argue that there is no such thing as an extended orgasm, that each time you go down, you end the orgasm. We believe that the coming-down phase of the orgasm is just as valid as the going-up part. We have pointed out that breaks between peaks can vary in length from a split second to minutes. At some point in going down, there comes a time when the orgasm stops, but this does not have to happen right away; the orgasm can last for a fairly long time on a downward ride.

By controlling when a person goes down, you are in a position to decide when to bring him or her back up. The ability to take someone up or down involves controlling the level of the tumescence; this is the essence of producing an EMO. It means you must be able to tell whether someone is going up or down, get into agreement with that direction, and make your next move accordingly.

Sensing the Energy

Down and *up* are, as we noted, just directions. They are "good" or "bad" only in relation to your goals. If you want to bring someone up and she comes down, that could be considered bad. If you want to bring someone down and he comes down, that could be considered good. The way you, the doer, can tell whether the doee goes down or up is by noticing how you feel. It is almost like an energy that you can sense in your body and mind. By focusing attention on this feeling, you start to notice the direction of the energy. You can even practice refining your up-and-down "meter" in everyday conversation—on the phone, in a classroom, or at work. Often, in conversations, the energy varies, sometimes moving up and at other times moving down. When the topic is titillating and fun—such as when you talk about sex or other exciting topics—you can notice the energy flowing upward. Then, when someone starts talking about a disease or about how he was mistreated, you

can notice the energy going downward. You do not even have to hear the words; you can simply feel it in your body.

We teach our DEMO class in three sessions. The morning is meant to tumesce the students slowly, bringing them higher and higher with peaks. We talk a lot about orgasm and other fun stuff. Then the second session is the orgasm itself. This takes everyone to the highest point before we begin to bring them down. The last session is informative, but it is also meant to gently bring everyone down to a much lower level of tumescence. We talk about topics such as safe sex and AIDS and other so-called negative subjects. We also peak the students a few times on the way down. Any non-English-speaker who was checking out the energy in the classroom could easily notice the varying energy levels. We deliberately vary energy levels, making them easy to notice; however, with proper attention, you can observe this sort of energy movement in everyday life.

Start noticing how you feel in relation to everyday activities. See if you can detect detumescence from your regular activities, such as eating or physical exercises that are known to detumesce people, such as yoga, weightlifting, or running. Massages and intercourse usually take their participants down very pleasurably. Intercourse usually involves a lot of physical pressure on both parties; they are banging against each other, and the male often ejaculates at the end. Some tumescence may occur, but—in the best scenarios—the end result is two pleasurably detumesced people.

Likewise, see if you notice any activities that tumesce you. Simply practice being aware of how you feel in relation to energy. Then the next time you are doing someone, you will be better able to trust your feelings about whether your partner is going up or down. In order to be good at noticing which way your partner goes, you have to take attention off of yourself and put it on your partner. Otherwise, what you are doing is similar to mental masturbation. There is a time and a place for that, too, but if you want to produce a great orgasm in someone, you must put your attention on that person. If you worry about how you are doing, why you are doing it, about the stock market, or about being victimized at work, the downward motion is self-propelled. You no longer notice your partner.

Sometimes, when a doee spaces out and no longer feels, the doer also spaces out and goes away. This is especially true for untrained doers. If you find yourself going away, it is time to come down and to take a break. It is time to talk about what is happening, because while you are talking you stay in present time and do not go away. To maintain control as a doer, it is best to realize that you've spaced out before your partner notices. If you do get caught, admit it and talk about what just happened, so that you can learn from it.

Controlling the Energy Through Intention

Putting all your attention on your partner enables you to be with him or her on every step of the orgasmic journey. Once you know which direction the energy is flowing, you can switch it seemingly at will by getting into agreement with the way it is actually going. You are not really switching it, but noticing that it is time to switch the direction. This lets your partner know that you're in control and will determine which way the energy flows. As long as the orgasm naturally keeps going higher, allow it to continue. Use your intention (which will be explained in more detail in the following paragraphs) to take the sensation up as far as it will go. The moment that you sense that it has stopped increasing—even before the orgasm starts to go down—is the best time to deliberately take it down; that way, you stay one step ahead. You will gain intuition from practice, and you will become better and better at knowing just when to peak your partner. This is the art of peaking, and, as we've said before, it is the basis of being able to create an EMO.

Using your intention during peaking is especially important. "Using your intention" means deciding firmly upon your purpose and focusing your attention accordingly. Your intention is your determination to act in a specified way. Although your intention involves firm decisions and specificity, you also must pay enough attention to notice when to change the intention—when to switch directions. Going down involves just as much attention as going up.

When the "going down" stage is temporary and you intend to take your partner up again, it's really not going all the way down—it's peaking. There are several ways to do this. A great way to very pleasurably bring a woman down a little is to make a long stroke all the way down her inner lips with one or two fingers, dip the fingers into her introitus, and stroke the fingers back upward toward her clitoris. She may be really high from the strokes on her clitoris, and this move enables her to catch up to the sensation and feel it all over her genitals. You can do the long stroke a few more times if it is a lot of fun. You can make the stroke as slow as you like. Then, when you go back to her clitoris, she will be able to go still higher. This is also a good way to lubricate the clitoris if it has begun to feel dry. The excess lubricant that you originally spread over her lips is available, and her introitus is probably somewhat wet from the clitoral stimulation.

Sometimes the doee, whether a man or a woman, is in such an excited state that he or she can hardly feel. In such a case, you actually can begin the do by deliberately taking your partner down a level or two so that he or she can feel more sensation. This may help your partner to relax. Before using any strokes to bring your partner up, apply firm pressure at any location on his or her body where you feel it will have the best effect. You can firmly press down with two hands, one on top of the other, on the abdomen. You can touch the forehead with one hand to get your partner back into the body. Pressing the sternum area, in the middle of the chest, can also be grounding. Do whatever it takes to help your partner feel more. If you notice that your partner is holding their breath or hyperventilating, ask them to take a few deep breaths and then to start breathing normally.

✒ Ejaculation ✑

The going-down part of the orgasm can be just as pleasurable, or more so, as the going-up; in fact, plenty of popular belief supports this notion. Ejaculation (see FIGURE 5.5, earlier) has been the stereotypical image people have of orgasm, but when a man starts ejaculating, he is actually on the way down. The tumescence builds until it bursts, and he ejaculates or explodes with release. Such an orgasm usually involves tenseness, and the person misses a lot of the pleasure on the way up so that he can experience the fun but short ride down. Although a person can experience a lot of pleasurable release on the way down, this traditional notion of the sensual experience is sort of like skiing: the uphill part of the experience happens only so we can have fun going downhill. With EMO, we can reverse directions—the going-up portion of the orgasm can be just as pleasurable as the going-down. A man needn't even ejaculate to have a great orgasm. This is what tantric sex is all about. Of course, we think it's unnecessary to give up ejaculation, especially if you can learn to appreciate the entire ride. Semen is mostly water and fructose and is easily regenerated. But it's important to learn to enjoy both sides of the mountain, for men as well as women—women can also feel a lot of sensation on the way down. Much energy can be released if a woman has gotten off well and her partner knows what to do to bring her down pleasurably.

✒ How Much Is Enough? ✑

A couple of questions that we hear often are "How do you know when to peak and dip your partner?" and "How do you know when to end the orgasm?" Let's address the second question first: the orgasm does not have to end when you stop stroking. Let us emphasize this point: *the orgasm ends when a person stops putting pleasurable attention on his or her own crotch.* We teach that on some level we are always in some form of orgasm—that we are coming all the time—but sometimes we notice it and other times we place our attention elsewhere. The orgasm is over when you have stopped noticing it.

You peak someone when you sense that he or she will no longer go higher. This sense is based on a feeling you get when you put your attention on someone else's orgasm. Sometimes you know it will be a quick dip and then off to the races again. Other times, you may be unsure whether your partner will go any higher. If you are unsure, then you are thinking about it, which means that your attention is already going down. When in doubt, *intend* for your partner to go down. There could still be more peaks later if you respond quickly. It is better to rub too little than too much. You know that it's time to stop stroking when you do not feel like stroking anymore.

DOWN AND UP AND UP AND DOWN You may decide to stop stroking because the peaks are no longer as much fun as they were before. It is best if you can realize this before it happens. This is quite difficult to do; even experts try to squeeze out one more peak when it's better to stop. The more you can tell when to quit the ride upward, the more control you have and the more your partner can surrender to you. When doing a woman, there comes a time when you try to give her an extra peak or two and she just doesn't go any higher. Simply point out to her that you thought she might go higher, but that you've since noticed that the highest point was one or two peaks ago. This shows her that you were there with her throughout the whole orgasm. It helps her to surrender to you the next time rather than wonder if you had spaced out. We recommend that people communicate with each other afterward to go over the experience. You can learn a lot by talking about the orgasmic experience after it happens.

Sometimes I tell the doee that this peak will be the last one. I may be teasing them, or I may feel that the doee has gone about as high as she is going to get this time out and I want to quit on the highest note. Sometimes the doee pleads with me to give her another peak or to continue to take her higher. If the pleading feels nongenuine, I say no. I can always peak her again to some extent on the way down (that technique is explained below). But if the pleading feels genuine—and not just because she thinks she *should* go higher—I offer to take her on another peak. I let her know that if she

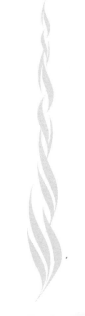

does not take it up quickly, I will stop. This could allow her to experience ever higher sensations.

If she fails to take it up quickly, I stop immediately and intentionally start to bring her down. I get to look good either way. If she goes up, she is happy, and the sensation for everyone increases. She gets to surrender more because she had to ask for more pleasure, and I'm a hero for taking her higher than either one of us thought she could get. On the other hand, if she fails to go higher, it shows that I was right to call the last peak the highest; this means she can trust my call more next time and therefore can surrender more easily.

If the doer tries to take the doee higher after the doer has sensed that their partner has reached the top, it can cause trouble. It may seem that the doer is going after the "success" of the experience, not the actual pleasure. You do not take someone higher by rubbing harder and faster (although that could be an occasional option) and by continuing despite all obstacles. Under these circumstances, the person getting rubbed goes numb and stops feeling. The person fails to pleasurably go up or down, because the doer is no longer acting deliberately. A doee will not surrender to a "bully" and will avoid repeating the experience. Doees want their partners to notice whether they are going up or down and to act accordingly. It is a delicate dance of awareness that demonstrates how much attention is focused upon the events at hand. As soon as the doee senses that he or she is no longer noticed, the doee stops feeling and takes back control of the nervous system. Let us repeat: if at any point you have doubt as to which direction the sensation is going, it is going down, so take a break and take it down deliberately. You can always go back up later.

Once you decide to take your partner down, you have lots of options. First you need to decide how fast or far to take your partner down, and whether you want to take your partner back up on the way down. To take someone back up after he or she has started to come down, all you have to do is start stroking again, using a steady reliable stroke; to have the intention to bring your partner back up; and to communicate what you are

FIGURE 10.1
Stroking the clitoris with palm on the mons area

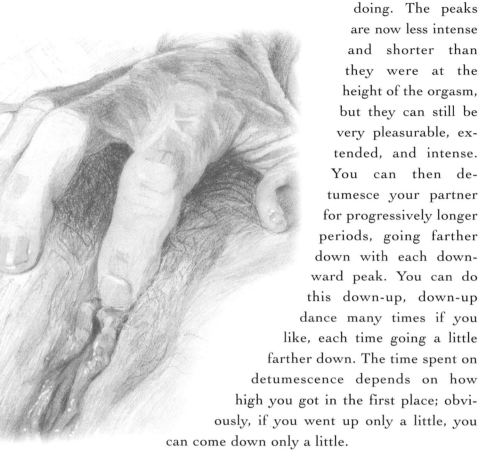

doing. The peaks are now less intense and shorter than they were at the height of the orgasm, but they can still be very pleasurable, extended, and intense. You can then detumesce your partner for progressively longer periods, going farther down with each downward peak. You can do this down-up, down-up dance many times if you like, each time going a little farther down. The time spent on detumescence depends on how high you got in the first place; obviously, if you went up only a little, you can come down only a little.

A fun stroke that we use to bring up a woman who's on the way down is to press the hand, palm down, on her mons area while stroking the clitoris with either the index or the middle finger (FIGURE 10.1). There's no need to anchor the clitoris, as it is still engorged and exposed. The pressure of the palm feels grounding, yet she goes up with the repeated stroke on the clitoris. This hand position can also be used on the way up, but because of the pressure involved, it works better on the way down. No matter what, it remains the intention of the doer that decides the direction in which the energy goes.

✐ Staying High ✐

Often people have only a limited amount of time for a sensual encounter, so they skip most of the ride down, except for the male squirting at the end. We recommend that you give the ride down at least an occasional visit. Sometimes it is fun to stay up and not come down at all, or to go only a little way down. Women seem to be more okay staying in this tumesced state. With proper training, men, too, can learn to feel comfortable without squirting and without needing to come down all the way. It is best to come down, at least to some extent, if you must go out in the world and need to do things such as drive a car. It's okay to stay up if you are at home and no worldly activities are calling you.

Women sometimes like to stay up after getting off and then use this elevated state to give their partners an orgasm. They may do their partners for a while and then have coitus, so they both can come down together. Other times, women just want to stay high and come down slowly, feeling the pleasure in their bodies for as long as possible. We know women who, after being done for an extended time, sometimes prefer not to go all the way down right away. They are able to feel pleasure and pulsations in their genitals for minutes or even hours after the last stroke. The amount of sensation you feel afterward depends on how high you were when you stopped and how much distraction confronts you. These women report that though the sensation slowly fades, if they put more attention on it, they can feel it more strongly and make it last longer. All that is necessary is relaxing and feeling the genitals. Eventually the sensations and pulsations stop, and the woman goes on to another activity.

Another reason to come down is that one or both of you may have something else to do. You can decide together beforehand that the orgasm will last fifteen minutes because that is all the time available at present. If one of you must go out and function in the world afterward, it is best that some of the time is spent coming down to a functional level.

✐ Deliberately Detumescing Your Partner ✐

"Detumescing" someone is the same as bringing them down. We repeat: you take someone down with intention. The best way to detumesce is by focusing your intention, increasing the pressure, and slowing down the stroke. You can, however, detumesce your partner with any stroke if your intention is strong enough. It is more your intention than the actual stroke that determines whether your partner goes up or down. With precisely the same stroke, you can bring your partner down if your intention is that she go down, or up if your intention is that she go up.

The best way to bring someone down quickly is with firm, usually incrementally increasing pressure. For a woman doee, place your palm over her pubic bone and press downward. Place your second hand on top of the first and press them down together (FIGURE 10.2). You can do a "pull-up": place the middle and ring fingers of either hand, pads up, inside the vagina and pull up on the pubic area while at the same time pushing down with the same palm on the outside of the pubic area. (FIGURE 10.3). You can also place your second hand on top of the first hand to add more pressure. The pressure forces the blood out of the genital area and brings her down quickly and pleasurably. You can also squeeze the clitoris through the hood between your thumb and index finger, which accomplishes the same goal (FIGURE 10.4).

She may or may not have strong contractions while you bring her down. These are still

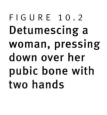

FIGURE 10.2
Detumescing a woman, pressing down over her pubic bone with two hands

part of the orgasm. Through them, she can release quite a bit of energy in a short time. Acknowledge any sensations you feel on the way down, just as you did on the way up. These may even be more intense than what you felt on the way up. The orgasm on the way down is just as valid as the one on the way up. It can feel great. It might even feel better. There is less pressure to perform, and she might be more relaxed. The main difference is that the energy level moves downward instead of upward.

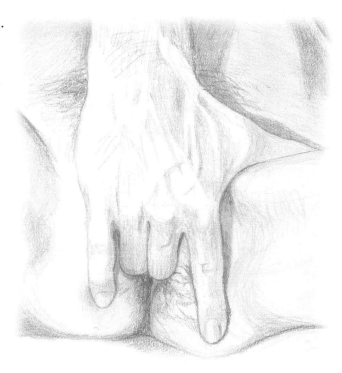

FIGURE 10.3
The "pull-up"

Some people enjoy harder pressure than others. Some may enjoy being whipped or spanked on the genitals or on the buttocks to bring them down. Slapping a woman's clitoris and vulva can be used, on rare occasions, to get her to feel more. Slapping the clitoris brings more

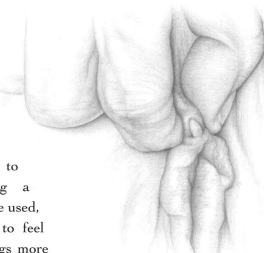

blood into the area and can be used as a kind of a jumpstart to take her up. It works by actually quickly bringing her down and thus allowing her to put her attention back on her pleasure when you return your finger to her clitoris. Avoid using this technique too often; it is not good for her to rely on the slap to be able to go up. Many people prefer not to be slapped at all, of course; you can use other techniques to peak them.

After a man ejaculates, he usually does not want to be touched directly on the penis, especially with firm pressure. The ejaculation itself, as we stated above, is already a detumescing act. You can put pressure on his abdomen, on his chest, right over his penis (on the mons area), on his upper thigh, or even on his forehead if you wish to bring him farther down. Pressing downward with one or both hands on any part of his body is detumescing if it's done with that intention. If the man does not ejaculate, you can apply firm pressure directly to his penis to intentionally bring him down. Intention is very important here, as squeezing the penis can take him up again if you are not careful.

Toweling Off

A nice way to end the orgasm is by toweling off. It brings a person farther down and also cleans up any lubricant. Check with your partner to find out how he or she likes to be toweled off. Most women seem to like a lot of pressure, and most men liked to be dabbed gently if they have ejaculated.

To towel off a woman, place a washcloth or a small hand towel, either folded in half or open, over her genitals. Using two to four fingers, firmly wipe off the excess lubricant. Start from the bottom of the perineum and slowly (take ten to thirty seconds) work your way up to above the clitoris (FIGURE 10.5). Stay in communication to determine the exact amount of pressure your partner prefers. It is always better to start lightly than to use too much pressure; it's better to incrementally increase your pressure than to work backward to less pressure.

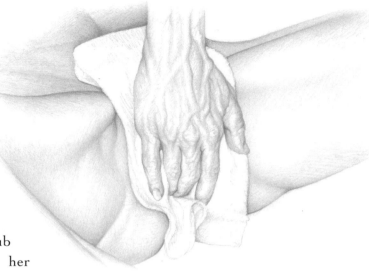

FIGURE 10.5
**Toweling off
a woman's
genitals**

Again,
you may
notice some
strong contrac-
tions as you rub
the towel along her
inner labia and over her
clitoris. This towel stroke can feel very pleasurable to her, as she continues to release energy on the way down.

The best way to towel off a man is to wipe away any excess lubricant and ejaculate
with a towel or
washcloth. Again,
it is probably best
to avoid placing
too much pressure
directly on the
penis. You can dab
the towel a num-
ber of times softly
against the penis
(FIGURE 10.6). You
can wrap the cloth
or towel around the

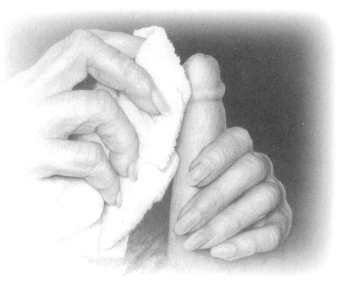

FIGURE 10.6
**Gently wiping
off the penis
with a towel**

FIGURE 10.7
Gently wrapping a towel around the penis to remove ejaculate and lubricant

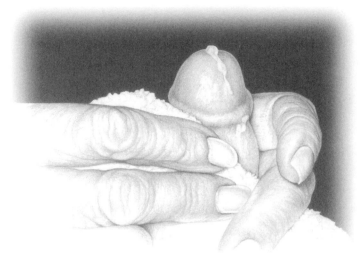

penis and lightly and slowly absorb the lubricant and semen (FIGURE 10.7). You can use more pressure on other parts of his genitals, such as his scrotum, perineum, and pubic hair, which might have a glob of ejaculate embedded in it. Communicate to find out exactly how your partner likes to be wiped dry.

We've come a long way, and this chapter has been a roller-coaster ride. We have come down, gone up, and come back down again. You'll discover that being in a detumesced state can increase your day-to-day functioning. You can make good decisions, and it takes more to stress you out. The world seems a better and brighter place after an EMO. You feel grounded, and things seem to run smoothly. Take a deep breath and enjoy the day.

~ Conclusion ~

No More Time
The fog dressed the castle,
With an invisible wand,
Waving her spell of forgotten night.
Once returned to her place,
Unveiled by reality's dream.
To soar as angels fly,
With wings so delicate,
With wings so sure,
With wings so light.
Unknown splendors,
Like a sorceress's delight.
The bed covered with sheets so white,
Of Egyptian cotton and virgin silk.
Pillows placed to support,
All of her charms,
Allowing movement,
Of her legs and arms.
Songs whistled in tones so pure,
Confidence sculpted by hands demure.
Shoulders bared, a kiss designed,
Taking care, so well defined,

Getting there in certain time,
Not ticking, for the magic rhyme
Will produce flowers instead of hours,
Lips that beckon, no fleeting second,
Tasty taste, no minutes to waste,
And candle's rays, no counting days

We have presented a lot of techniques and information. They are, of course, important to absorb and learn if you are going to become a serious sensual student. But we also want to make it clear that fun and playfulness are even more important than all the techniques we've presented. You will become proficient at the techniques with enough practice. Those practice sessions don't have to be difficult or scary. Don't get upset if you are not the world's best doer the first few times you try. You would not expect to be a world-class tennis player after reading a book and practicing a couple of times. You don't have to be a superb athlete or have musician's hands in order to be a wonderful giver or receiver of an EMO. Appreciate any improvement that you do make. If you used to have a ten-second orgasm and now it lasts twenty seconds, you have improved by 100 percent. You will be amazed at how quickly you are able to extend your orgasm—if you do not get impatient or upset. The intensity of the orgasm may at first seem even less than what you are used to. Again, with a little patience and practice, the intensity will increase dramatically.

Although penises and clitorises have been around forever, the techniques and information on how to create an EMO have been around for only about twenty-five years, since the last quarter of the twentieth century. Because it is such a new discipline, there are many opportunities to further develop and create new ways and styles to take the art of orgasm even higher. With practice and deliberate training, you can become a virtuoso and create new styles and new strokes of your own.

Of the billions of people in the world, only a very small percentage presently are able to experience either giving or receiving an EMO. We believe that people who are able to push the envelope and give sensuality a high priority in their lives will make their own lives, as well as the lives of the people around them, better and more fun. People who experience EMOs and know that they can have a great orgasm or can produce a great orgasm at will walk around with more confidence in all aspects of their lives. They do not feel needy and are able to express themselves with more generosity. Most people are unaware of the amazing potential that the human nervous system has to experience EMOs. As we have stated, you do not have to have any special abilities to learn to give or receive an EMO. All you need to have is the desire, and all you need to do is follow the instructions that we have laid out for you.

We also feel that you deserve to be congratulated for having read this book and making sensuality and pleasure a higher priority in your life. It is not easy to go for pleasure, and your decision to do so has taken a certain amount of courage and guts. Our egos do not like to admit that there may be something to learn about sexuality, and they feel threatened when we do open up to this possibility. We judge ourselves very heavily on our ability to be good in bed, and we do not like to consider the possibility that, actually, we may not know that much. Once we do open up and admit that there may be something to learn, we reap many rewards. Of course, the more you practice the techniques and information that we have described, the more your life will benefit. When our egos have learned a powerful lesson, our lives become that much better.

Having sex or a sensual experience is best when it is accompanied by real desire, although one does not have to wait till one is totally filled with passion and lust. You could do it just because you think that it is a good idea, or because there is nothing else that you would rather do. Once one starts, the desire usually comes along too. A sensual experience is also not something that you *have* to do. It is not like eating and drinking: if you don't eat or drink, you will get sick and eventually die. You can go without sex, obviously, for a long time, and if you do not feel compelled to engage in it, you should not beat yourself over the head because you think that you should have it.

We think that the information in this book is valuable to people of all ages. There is a new trend in colleges and universities that's called "hooking up." It is actually similar to the "one-night stand," which has been around for many years. Hooking up involves having casual sex with someone you either don't know very well or someone with whom you don't want a relationship. Hooking up is done by many people in their late teens and early twenties. We do not think that it is harmful, per se, for young people to explore their sensuality and sexuality. Some of these people report that they kiss and "make out" but do not go all the way. Others state that they go all the way and that they do it with more than one person. The harm or danger comes from having unprotected intercourse. Even when using condoms, there is still a significant risk that some accident, such as a venereal disease or a pregnancy, could result. The cure for HIV/AIDS has not yet been discovered and may never be. We think that people have intercourse because they don't know of a better way to have intimacy and pleasure. Learning about EMOs can be a good solution for younger people.

The ability to create an orgasm in your partner by hand is also a wonderful gift for older people. Many older men cannot have erections as they did when they were younger. They occasionally get hard, but many report that they get only somewhat engorged; the penis is heavy yet not fully erect. Many older women lose vaginal lubrication (they get less "wet") as they age. A not fully erect penis inserted into a dry vagina has a poor chance of being very pleasurable for either party. The use of our hands, with either a water-soluble or insoluble lubricant, upon the genitals of our partners is about pure pleasure, with no performance anxiety. We can rub our partners for an extended amount of time, whether the penis is erect or not, whether the vagina is wet or not.

Take whatever works for you from this book. It is not meant to replace communication but to open up communication and bring it to a new and higher level. If the words we use or suggest that you say while you're having or giving an EMO seem awkward or silly, replace them with your own. They are only examples and ideas that have aided some of our students and ourselves. They are not written on stone, only on paper.

The information in this book also is meant to add to whatever sex life you already have. These techniques and tips are things that you *can* do, not things that you *should* do. We don't want you to give anything up that you are enjoying now. We have written this book with the strict intention of showing how to create intense orgasmic pleasure in one's partner through a hand-to-genital method. This does not mean that we think people should give up romance, cuddling, or any type of genital contact. As we described in the "Teasing" chapter, you don't start a sensual experience with the genitals; you get there only if both partners are aroused and interested. It may seem that we get to the genitals quite quickly in this book, and that has been deliberate due to the techniques we discuss.

There are parts of this book that we highly recommend for improving almost everyone's sex life. For example, getting the woman engorged before intercourse is just as necessary as getting the man engorged. We suggest other techniques—such as spanking and slapping—that do not necessarily have to be used in order to have a fantastic sex life. You will learn what you like, and hone your skills, by reading this book. However, most of the information has to be incorporated and practiced regularly if you want to take your sex life to a new and more intense level. Just reading this book doesn't make you a better lover. You have to read it and then apply the various techniques and communication skills till they are part of you.

When we give our students homework—practicing the masturbation exercises or having their partners give them an orgasm—they almost always do the assigned tasks. They have paid quite a bit of money, they have peer pressure from classmates, and they deliberately have taken time to enhance their sex lives. You've paid only the price of this book, and there is no peer pressure around to make you want to practice. You have, however, taken the time to read this book, and the best way to incorporate its information is to practice its techniques with as much enthusiasm as you can. Do the masturbation exercises often. Do them because it feels good and because you want to learn more about your body. You can always find something new and wonderful about your body that you can then bring into your love life. Teach your partner, if you have one, about your body and how best to touch it. One of the best ways to learn to have an EMO is to give one to someone else, and vice versa. Find out how your partner likes to be touched, and practice giving him or her orgasms, too. Learn how much fun you can have giving, as well as receiving, an EMO. If you do not have a regular partner, you can find either a romantic partner or a partner who just wants to do research with you.

In our many years of teaching, we have noticed that sometimes when women find out how much fun they can have with manual clitoral stimulation, they take a break from wanting to play with a man's genitals. They may feel that their clitoris and orgasm have been neglected for so long that now they cannot get enough of their pleasure. We recommend to their male partners that they not get angry or stop rubbing on these women. After enough attention, women feel filled up and feel more inclined to start playing with a man's private parts again. And when they do, it is with a new appreciation and generosity. These women don't touch men because they feel they have to or to get them off their backs but because they genuinely want to, because they desire "cock." We also tell these women that the more generous they are in doling out pleasure to their men, the more pleasure they can have and receive. To have an EMO, it's very helpful if you are able to give one. If you are unwilling to give someone your undivided attention, you will probably doubt their sincerity in wanting to give you theirs. This doubt is an obstacle in your ability to surrender to their touch and attention. You will see their attention as either manipulative or as a tit-for-tat exchange, and that will prevent you from "giving it up" to them.

Another—and nonsexual—way that a number of students have opened themselves to having more pleasure in their lives is by doing anonymous good deeds. People's ability to have pleasure is somehow correlated with how

good they feel about themselves. When a person does something nice for someone else, or even for an animal or a plant, and does it in a way that is anonymous, the person usually feels better about herself. It can be nice to do or give something to another human being, but if it is not anonymous, it is more like a trade than a gift. It can still help you feel good and better about yourself, but this "trade" doesn't have as much impact as a gift given in secret.

Although you have almost finished reading this book, your work is far from over, if you can call it work. You now can apply what you have learned. Keep this book nearby, as you cannot be expected to remember everything you have read; then you can later review parts that come up in your sex life. Read it with your partner, or give your partner a copy of their own. If you do have any specific questions that we did not cover in this book, email us. They could be the basis for our next book. Our e-mail address is verasteve@aol.com.

— Ideas for —
Communication

ACKNOWLEDGMENTS FOR THE DOEE ⤳ Here are some examples of things the doee can say to acknowledge the doer.

Wow!

That feels great!

So good.

You are the best.

Great hands.

Yes!

Oh, my!

Oh, God!

You got me good.

That's terrific.

Fantastic!

The best yet.

I feel so high!

Your finger on my spot feels delicious.

I can feel the sensation spread down my legs to my toes.

It's spreading up my torso, into my arms, and out my fingers.

You are so sexy!

I love your thighs.

I love your body.

You have sexy arms.

Wonderful touch!

Love your hands.

That's even better!

That's it!

You're on my spot.

Perfect pressure!

ACKNOWLEDGMENTS FOR THE DOER Here are some examples of things the doer can say to acknowledge the doee.

You feel so good!

Good girl or Good boy. *[Avoid sounding sexist.]*

You are turning me on.

You are getting me hard.

Touching your penis makes my pussy feel sensational.

You feel great!

It's so much fun to do you.

You are such a pleasure to touch.

Great contractions!

Sweet pussy!

Great cock!

You respond so well to directions.

Or try any of the positive things listed below in "Reporting What You Notice," or anything listed above in "Acknowledgments for the Doee" (use "genitals" instead of "hands").

COMMANDS FOR THE DOER ⤳ Here are some examples of commands or requests that the doer can use to get the doee to feel more. It is important to always let the doee know right away when they have succeeded even a little bit.

Take it higher.

Take it up.

Give me more.

Fill the room.

Have the neighbors feel it.

Give it up!

Relax.

Relax your anus.

Relax your face.

Push out.

Feel 15 percent more.

Feel my finger.

Feel the next stroke.

Take it to the next level.

Lie still.

Melt into the bed.

Sink into my hand.

REPORTING WHAT YOU NOTICE, FOR THE DOER Here are some examples of phrases the doer can use to report any signs of orgasm and anything else he or she notices in the doee.

I can feel you getting harder.

You are getting more engorged.

Your introitus is wet.

The sensation is building.

Your clitoris feels electric.

Your coming is easy.

Your pussy [penis] looks beautiful!

Your clitoris is twice its normal size.

Your clitoris is totally exposed from its hood.

Your genitals are turning redder.

Your balls have [scrotum has] moved toward your body.

Your face and neck are flushed.

I can smell your semen.

The head of your cock just got bigger.

I can feel you going up!

I can feel you coming down!

You are really relaxed.

This is the highest so far!

Your contractions are getting stronger.

You have strong ridging [or contractions] in your abdomen.

— Commonly Asked — Questions and Answers

The questions we received from readers of our first book, *Extended Massive Orgasm,* determined much of the shape and content of this book. Here are other questions we commonly hear. We hope our responses assist you in your study and practice of EMO.

Q I find vaginas to be very different from one another, though most men say that women are all the same down there. I've observed very big clitoral differences. They can be tiny; they can be huge. Do you, Vera and Steve, think that some vaginas are more orgasmic then others? Do you think the size of the clitoris is important to the "quality" of the orgasm?

A Vaginas are not orgasmic; what makes some vaginas seem to be the source of orgasm is their position in relation to the clitoris (read more about this in Chapter 9). Every woman's genitals are unique in terms of their size and shape; no two women are alike (except maybe identical twins). The size of the clitoris, in general, does not affect the intensity or duration of the orgasm. Women with clitorises ranging in size from small to extra-large can experience an EMO. Some clitorises, however, are difficult to reach. Either the hood won't retract, or the clitoris is so small you can hardly feel it. It may be difficult to give such women an EMO. However, with enough love and attention, you can learn how best to stimulate these women. In fact, we have even seen clitorises get larger with use.

Q Speaking about sizes, here's an eternal male question—am I big enough? Most men would rather have a huge penis than a huge brain. What would you, Vera and Steve, say to those guys?

A First of all, just having a larger brain doesn't necessarily make you smarter. And having a larger penis definitely does not make you any smarter, or a better lover. Penises come in all sizes; moreover, some men with small penises have a large coefficient of expansion (meaning that their penises grow quite a bit when erect), and others with large penises have a small coefficient of expansion (meaning that they grow only somewhat when erect). When men are together in a locker room, they think the man with the largest penis has something they don't have. But the women we know really don't care. They may say things to hurt a man if he believes he is too small, but in truth it really doesn't matter to them. As we wrote in our last book, once a woman is engorged and pushed out, a thumb inserted just a half-inch can feel like six or more inches of penetration (see Chapter 6 of this book for a description of the push out). Penis size has no bearing on the sensual satisfaction of a woman in this condition. If a man is ignorant about how to pleasurably engorge a woman before inserting his penis, a larger one might make more contact—but this should only concern guys who are poor at pleasing a woman; and with willingness, training, and enthusiasm, even they can learn to do it better. We think an old Tibetan saying is apropos here: "If you find yourself in the body of a donkey, enjoy the grass." Find the penis size that you were blessed with a true blessing, enjoy who you are, and learn how to use your hands.

Q How can I get my wife to try your techniques? She resists doing anything new, especially in bed.

A You first have to believe that who she is and what she does is okay. People refuse offers if they somehow feel that they would lose if they were to accept the offer. Your wife may think you are dissatisfied with who she is and what she does, that you want her to be different and to change. People are also afraid to try something new if they fear they won't be good at it. Sometimes people get into habits and will do something different only when the habit causes them too much discomfort. But even with discomfort, breaking negative habits can be a challenge; we have known a number of people with emphysema who tried to give up smoking cigarettes, but couldn't. Your wife may also refuse your advances because she is pissed at you for any number of past occurrences.

You will be most likely to get her to try something different if you first get in agreement with her viewpoints. Try to understand—without probing for answers—why she might resist your advances. Also, women love flattery; you can tell her how beautiful and sexy she is many times before she has heard enough. Notice what you like and love about her and communicate that, whether it is her smooth skin, her beautiful eyes, or her sense of humor.

Tell yourself that you're playing a game—the game of seduction. You win at this game when everyone is happy and you accomplish your goal—or at least move in the direction of your goal. The goal here is to get your wife to play with some new techniques and sensual ideas. The bigger the obstacle in a game, the more valuable the goal becomes. The more resistance there is to overcome, the more you value the result you achieve. If someone offers no resistance, the game would be too easy, and reaching your goal would hold little value. There would be no game if there were no resistance.

When you are seducing someone, you are playing with their viewpoints and emotions. Therefore, proceed with respect and resist getting argumentative. To be good at seduction, you must focus a lot of attention on the other person. You must notice when they are coming toward you and when they are going away. Another name for this game is "push/pull." When someone is going away, it is best to push them even farther and faster away than they are willing to go on their own. When someone is coming toward you, make them offers and pull them closer—and it's even better if they believe it was their intention, rather than your scheming, that reeled them in. Whichever direction you're moving, the most important part is to enjoy the seduction. Make it a fun game for you and for her. If you enjoy yourself, she will appreciate your attention.

So, in order to make this a game, first *agree* with your wife's resistance to trying new techniques. You can even think up reasons why it wouldn't be a good idea. Talk through these reasons with her. Here are some possible reasons to try out. (Again, each person is different, and these are only examples that may or may not work with your particular partner.)

1. She might become addicted to sex. She may like it so much that she loses her job.

2. It is best not to change one's mind once it is made up.

3. Her whole value system may become skewed; she won't be the same person anymore.

4. You may lose your job because she wants to do it all the time.

5. Your family may starve, because the two of you will forget about eating.

6. If the neighbors knew, they would think you are weird.

7. She might start to really like you, and then she wouldn't get to argue or fight with you anymore.

After bringing up each reason, give her the opposite reason, explaining why these ideas are not really true. This enables you to inform her about why, in reality, reasons for not doing it are invalid. This is where knowing your partner and focusing attention on her pay off. The more attention you pay to her and the better you know her, the more you know what to say to her and when to say it.

This is how you seduce someone. You push and then you pull. You take away and then you give. Without touching her, you are already doing her mind, so you are in essence already using the new techniques on her. If you continue the seduction, there will come a point when you feel her resistance wane. You can then grab her hand and lead her to the bedroom. Explain that you will only do it for, say, five minutes. And when those five minutes are up, don't continue. It is better to do less and to leave her wanting more. Most men, when they finally get their partners to agree to try new techniques, tend to do too much and to be so concerned with the success of the experience that they miss the best time to stop.

Q I was doing my girlfriend, and midway through the experience she started to shake all over. Is that part of the orgasm? What was happening?

A The shaking and spasms you observed in your girlfriend are not part of the orgasm but are actually symptomatic of a body that is unused to a certain level of intensity and has become uncomfortable. The tremors are a sign that the body is resisting the orgasm; they occur when the person is tense instead of relaxed. (Note, too, that men as well as women can exhibit tension through shaking and spasms.) So they are, on one hand, a good sign because you probably took her to a level of intensity that she had not experienced before, or at least not very often. However, if you wish to take her even higher, you want her to be as relaxed as possible (without falling asleep).

You might have noticed that she tensed up before the tremors even started. The more practiced you are and the more attention you focus on her—skills that will develop naturally with additional experience—the better able you are to determine her state of tension. The next time she starts shaking, you will know to stop and take a break. Let her know that you are having fun and that she really is doing well and feeling a lot. Tell her that you want her to relax, and that if you feel her tense up when you continue stroking, you will remind her to relax. Tell her that she does not have to do anything to relax—she just needs to hear the suggestion and her body automatically will become more relaxed.

In order to feel the most intensity—in order to experience a massive orgasm—it is paramount to sink into the bed and relax. We sometimes help our students to relax by suggesting an analogy: "Feel like a pad of butter melting in the sunlight." We also tell them to relax their anuses. The relaxation of the anus causes them to relax their whole genital area. We ask our female students to push out and then to relax. Sometimes I put my finger inside the introitus and ask her to push my finger out and then to relax. We do whatever it takes to help the person relax.

Q   I met this really nice woman who likes to have sex. The only problem is that her pussy smells bad. Do you recommend that I tell her, and if so, how?

A   This is a delicate situation, but it does require a solution. She obviously does not know that her genitals smell bad, or she would have dealt with the problem—both women and men, were they aware they had such a problem, would attempt to fix it. There could be a number of reasons for the problem. She could have a yeast infection or an STD. Yeast infections usually are associated with a whitish discharge from the vagina. If there is any discharge or sores associated with the smell, do not go any further; instead, recommend that she seek medical attention. More likely, however, she just employs poor hygiene down there. And sometimes the smell may actually be caused by fear and apprehension. With loving attention and some stroking, such smells often miraculously disappear. But whatever the cause, she'd benefit from your telling her about the problem.

When training someone in EMOs, it is always best to start with positive comments. Therefore, before you blurt out that her "pussy stinks," tell her how beautiful her pussy is or make any other approving remarks. You then can let her know, tactfully, that an odor is emanating from her genitals. If it is really offensive, you could suggest that she go to the bathroom and wash up. When she returns, let her know that the smell is gone. We have been amazed at the poor hygiene exhibited by many new students. We have seen many a crusty crotch, and in those cases we ask the students to clean up. Many people in Europe have a bidet, which is an excellent tool for cleaning the genitals. But a regular shower, with soap and water and thorough washing, usually does the trick. We do not think douching is a good idea, unless the hygiene is terribly offensive.

Finally, be aware that there is a difference between a strong but fragrant genital odor and a foul-smelling one. The more turned on a woman is, the more you will enjoy everything about her, including whatever smells she may have.

In any case, your girlfriend most likely will appreciate that you had the guts to bring up the taboo subject of her smelly crotch and will be glad to clean up. She might be embarrassed at first but probably will be thankful later. There is a small chance that she might be so offended that she will break up with you. However, she probably will correct the problem anyway, and she'll be better off because of you.

Q You teach mostly couples who already have good sex lives. Why do you feel it's important to teach them to improve their sex lives, particularly through extended massive orgasm?

A We teach anyone who comes to us with the desire to improve their lives. We teach not only couples but also single people who want more fun in their lives. We are not therapists, and if people think they have a physical or mental problem, we send them to a doctor or therapist. Although it is true that we prefer to teach people who already have great sex lives and are looking for ways to enhance them, we also teach people who have had very little sex or very few orgasms before they met us. We have taught a number of male virgins who are now very popular with the ladies. We have taught many women who thought they could not have an orgasm, and we have shown them how they could—and they always have.

The reason we prefer to teach people who already enjoy a good sex life is that we can take them even higher than they've gone in the past. Teaching is most fun when people are going for excellence. It is easy to go from bad to good or okay, because the past history that you call "bad" chases you and prods you to improve. But when you start from a place that is already good and you want to go to better still, you have only yourself and your desires to lead you there. There is nobody and nothing chasing you.

Both Vera and I enjoy this line of work. We both enjoy watching people flash to new viewpoints, and our ability to help others exponentially increase their orgasmic potential is very rewarding to us. We both love to see women go for their own pleasure and become freer people. What could be more fun work than playing with a woman's genitals and making it an educational experience? And our own sex life keeps expanding as a byproduct of giving others this wonderful information. One of the best ways to get better at something, and to have more of it in your life, is to teach it.

Q Vera, obviously you are a very sexual and very orgasmic woman. When did you become aware of this? What do you feel when you are coming and coming? How do you feel afterward?

A The answer starts in my childhood. I was living at a displaced person's camp in Salzburg after World War II. My mother and I were in a concentration camp for a year before that because she belonged to the resistance in Yugoslavia. I was ten or eleven years old. There were very narrow hallways in our building. One day, I was walking down the hallway and an elderly man who had visited a neighbor was heading toward me. We stopped, and he put his hand directly on my clitoris through my dress. I do not know if he knew exactly where he was touching me, but I felt a sudden burst of pleasure. He removed his hand after a few seconds and went on his way. After this episode I began to play with myself and feel my own clitoris.

The first time I had a real sexual experience was with a tennis instructor at a summer camp in Austria. I was fifteen and was flashing him in my bikini. He became upset with me and followed me into a dressing room. He spanked me and then sucked on my genitals. I felt great pleasure, and I consider this my first orgasm.

To answer your second question: During orgasm my attention is on the pleasure that my body experiences. I remain as relaxed as I can in order to feel the most. It is difficult to describe this pleasure, but I will do my best. It is as though waves of sensation are pulsing through my entire body. My clitoris feels the most sensation, but I also feel these waves coming down into me through my head, into my body, down my legs and arms, and out through my fingers and toes. This is continuous and repeats over and over. My abdomen ridges and pulses, and there are continuous contractions in my vagina and entire vulval area that feel wonderful. It is kind of an electricity moving through my genitals and body. It is like being covered by an ocean of pure joy in which the waves get bigger and bigger, flatten out when I'm being peaked, and then get higher and higher once the stimulation starts again.

The finger on my clitoris feels like it is touching and highlighting the center of my being, making me feel totally alive, the source of all this magnificent intense sensation. I can feel any contact with my partner's body—the remarkable hand inside my vagina finding new places of pleasure, or a hand on my breast or wherever—as an addition to the pleasure originating from that most sensational organ, my clitoris.

After it is done, I feel refreshed. I feel wonderful all over. My body is glistening, and I can tell that my face is glowing. My awareness is heightened. Food tastes better; flowers smell more delicious. Life is more blissful.

Q And, Steve, do you regard yourself a very sexual person?

A I consider myself a very sensual person. I love being turned on by a woman, whether she has use for my penis, she is flirting, or she is just testing her equipment. When I lived communally, during our years at university, I rubbed on and gave great orgasms to as many women as possible. This was fun, and also educational. When we started a sensuality department at the commune/university, I did what it took to become a teacher in the program so I could expand my knowledge of sensuality as well as increase the variety of women and kinds of pleasure I experienced. Although I was married to Vera, I had a number of girlfriends at the commune and usually said yes to any offers they made, as long as Vera approved. Vera was there for some of these activities and passed on being there for others. I have always masturbated, and with the information learned through years of my sensual training, this too has gotten better. Before the onset of the HIV/AIDS epidemic, I experienced all kinds of sexual activities, although most of them involved hand-to-genital stimulation. Since the epidemic began, I engage only in hand-to-genital contact, except with Vera. Now that we live by ourselves, we have a wonderful and intimate sex life with each other.

Q Vera, part of your degree requirements involved coming for three hours in front of your professors. Can you describe it? How was it for you?

A It was an intense experience. This was a test I had to pass in order to become part of the faculty and to teach for my school. It was fun, but not the most fun I have experienced. The teacher who gave me the orgasm was not someone I now consider to be a great sexer. When Steve rubs on me for three hours, which he has done a number of times, it is much more fun than that experience was, and I can go higher.

The experience was very clinical, but when I am having an orgasm, my attention is on what I feel, not on my surroundings. My orgasm keeps getting better with time and practice; my degree test happened in 1980, so it was not as good as what I can experience now, twenty-plus years later.

Q What is your opinion on quickies? I mean, sometimes there is no time for long sessions, and sometimes there is nothing better than a quickie (my wife agrees).

A We think quickies are great! A person can be gratified with just a few moments of directed pleasure. When a person can get off starting with the first stroke, every stroke is orgasmic. We have done sessions with students in which we tell them in advance that they will get only one stroke. They put all their attention on that stroke, and, many times, it becomes one of their most memorable experiences. Most other primates—and other animals, for that matter—have intercourse that lasts only a few seconds. So if you have only a few minutes before having to be somewhere or do something, it can be very invigorating and gratifying to have a quickie.

Q I have a question that's prompted by the huge publicity fellatio has received, thanks to Bill and Monica! How important is fellatio to you, Steve? Could fellatio be overrated (like the band U2, who are very good, but still not as good as they're made out to be)? And Vera, how important is cunnilingus to you?

A Using the tongue can be very erotic. However, you can employ your finger with much more precision than your tongue. Would you want a brain surgeon to go into your head with his tongue, his penis, or his hand? Vera enjoys cunnilingus, but it is more of an erotic thrill than a means to the best orgasm. If a woman is healthy and smells great, it can be fun and exciting to lick and suck on her pussy. It also tastes great, and these additional senses can add to the experience. I love licking and sucking on Vera, but I don't do it with others; because of the possibility of disease, we think oral sex is best done between longtime partners.

I have enjoyed fellatio, too, depending on who was doing it. On rare occasions, I have been done by a woman who really liked sucking cock, and this was most enjoyable. But most of the time I prefer that the woman use her hands rather than her mouth. Again, with fellatio there is a greater chance of spreading disease, and, since one of the participants has her (or his) mouth full, the communication is poorer, and that's detrimental to a great experience. I have often found that a woman will put her partner's penis in her mouth just so she doesn't have to talk.

The combination of a hand or both hands with a mouth on a penis can be extremely sensational if done properly. The drawback is finding a lubricant that the woman doesn't mind getting in her mouth. (We have added flavorings to lubricants to make them taste better.) I also enjoy it when a woman uses her whole arm, leg, breast, foot, or another part of her anatomy in combination with her hands on my penis, as long as she is touching me for her own pleasure.

Q Do you believe that there are women who need ages to come and women who cannot come at all? What advice would you offer to these unhappy ladies? Should they keep trying to catch an orgasm, or let the orgasm catch them?

A When most people talk about women taking ages to come, they usually mean that these women take a long time to come during *intercourse.* Actually, most women are unable to come during intercourse, and even the ones that can don't every time. This is because there are no nerve endings on the vaginal wall. Some women's clitorises are closer to their vaginal opening than others'; if it's close enough, the clitoris can be stimulated by the movement of the penis. Other women have built a connection between their vaginal opening and their clitoris and are therefore more orgasmic with penetration. (See the "Connections" exercise in the "Masturbation" chapter for information on building connections.)

We have found that all women are orgasmic with clitoral stimulation. Some women are more orgasmic or seem to come more easily and intensely than others. But all healthy women who have made this type of sensual stimulation a priority in their lives can experience an orgasm from the first stroke and can learn to intensify their orgasms with practice. So even if she is not very orgasmic at first, a woman can learn to become very sensual and sensitive. Of course, there are differences among all women; some may take to our techniques like a duck to water, and others may need more swimming lessons.

We suggest that people have intercourse only when they really want to. We urge women and men to learn more about clitoral stimulation—what strokes, pressures, and speeds feel best—and to learn how to communicate their preferences to their partners.

Q   What are the differences between men's and women's desires in bed?

A   Most people think that men just want to have sex and care for little else, while women want love and affection. This apparent difference is caused by the fact that most people use the word *sex* to mean *intercourse*. When men have intercourse, they usually have an orgasm, but most women do not. Besides being less pleasurable for women, intercourse is riskier for them, too; they're the ones who get pregnant, and women may be more vulnerable to some STDs, such as HIV. Many women fake their pleasure; they have intercourse as a way to either get the man off their back (or front) or to get something in return from him. (A woman doing the latter is actually dealing sex, not enjoying it; see Helen Fisher's book *The Sex Contract.*)

In reality, women want pleasure just as much, if not more, than men do. And their bodies are designed for it: the clitoris is the only organ on a human being that has the sole function of pleasure.

A woman who knows what she likes and is willing to communicate it to her partner is a gratified woman. But, for the best results, she must communicate her desires in a nice way. Men love to win and succeed. If a woman lets her partner know when he is doing well, rather than telling him he's messing up again, he is much more interested in listening to her. Then, once she has gotten his ear, she can tell him exactly what she would like. Men can be slow to figure out what women are actually saying, so a woman gets the best results when she is exact and precise in her communications. (The word *nice*, in fact, used to mean "precise.") If the man still does not understand precisely what a woman wants, she should repeat herself in exactly the same way until he gets it (and, ultimately, she gets it).

A woman who is familiar with her clitoris and its capabilities is in a great position to teach her partner about it. Most men know very little about the clitoris, but once they find out about it, they want to become proficient at touching and stimulating it. Many women who have learned to experience wonderful orgasms through clitoral stimulation no longer fear sexual intimacy with men. These women are just as willing to have fun in bed as men are. These women are turned on and are at least, if not more, orgasmic than men. They are gratified sexually and get the love and attention and affection they desire.

To these women and their partners, sex is no longer just about intercourse. It is about sensuality, pleasure, fun, and great communication. A woman who knows what she wants and is willing to express it will see her desires manifested. We had a friend who liked a new man. She wanted to have fun with him but didn't want to have intercourse. They kissed for almost four hours, and the man was thrilled about it. He felt like a winner and did not think he had missed out on anything. These gratified women do not condemn intercourse, but if they do have it, they are sure to derive pleasure from it. This usually means they desire orgasmic stimulation of the clitoris before any penetration with the engorged penis. Men who learn to pleasure and gratify women are valued lovers. They learn how to communicate about giving and receiving pleasure. They become more confident lovers, and more confident people in all other aspects of their lives.

Bottom line: Both sexes desire fun and pleasure in bed, and when they learn how to give and receive the gifts of sensual awareness and satisfaction, both become more confident and gratified overall.

Q Steve, can you describe your technique for stroking the clitoris?

A Detailing our methods is what this book and our last one are all about. Basically, I take pleasure from touching the clitoris, which I consider to be the most fun organ in all of creation. I worship it. There are always new, fun strokes and ways to touch the clitoris that I learn each time I have a chance to get my fingers on one. I really enjoy teasing it, getting it to stand on its hind legs, so to speak, and beg to be touched. I enjoy making it come out to attack my finger for its own greedy gratification.

Q Since Freud's dismissal of the clitoral orgasm as inferior and his claim that the vaginal orgasm was superior—and especially after the G-spot was discovered—there has been big debate about which of the two is the better, stronger orgasm. Your comment? Which is your favorite coital position? Which is the most "orgasmic"?

A As we have said, all orgasm is clitorally based. Even the G-spot is formed of the lower part, or roots, of the clitoris and its innervating nervous system. The vaginal wall contains no nerve endings for touch and pleasure. It is homologous in embryology to the male scrotal sac. Therefore, as far as sensation goes, there is no comparison between the clitoris and the vagina, as the clitoris has approximately eight thousand nerve endings on it. The apex of the male penis has about ½ as many nerve endings.

Our favorite coital position is what we call the conversational position. We lie side by side, and our legs are intertwined and can move around. We can talk and kiss. We like other positions, too, especially the woman on top. We emphasize, however, that each couple prefers different positions; it is up to each to find the best, most orgasmic positions for themselves. We are not experts in intercourse, but we do believe it is important for both partners to be engorged and to desire insertion before penetration occurs.

Q How often do you, Steve and Vera, have sex? Do you agree with me in saying that couples should try to have sex at least once a day?

A First of all, I (that's me, Vera, speaking) do not like the word *should*. So when you say couples "should" have sex once a day, it makes me cringe. Sometimes we have sex daily, sometimes we may skip a few days, and sometimes we have sex or give each other orgasms many times during the day. We are fortunate in that we have arranged our lives so that we are together almost all the time; we have no children living with us, and we can do pretty much whatever we please. We are nice to each other, are romantic, hug every few hours at least, and kiss each other numerous times throughout the day. We think it is valuable to be intimate with your partner; having sex or giving your partner a great orgasm is very beneficial in becoming closer, having fun, and being thrilled with your life.

It is helpful to deliberately plan times when you can be alone with your partner and have this kind of intimacy. This does not rule out spontaneity, but if you base your sex life on spontaneity, you may never get there. The more deliberately you plan for pleasure, the more pleasure you'll receive. So if you have small children, have someone take care of them for an evening, and go to a hotel. Do what you need to in order to be alone with your partner.

As part of their homework, we recommend to students that they have one, two, or more orgasms each day. A woman who can have an EMO no longer has to be concerned or have anxiety about her ability to experience her sexual potential. She is at peace or in agreement with her sexual capacity and no longer feels as though she is lacking anything sexually. Many of our students, however, continue getting off daily even though it is no longer mandatory. Here's the key: Do only what you really want to do. You do not have to have sex to be a good person. If there is something you find objectionable but still feel you have to do, then change your mind about how objectionable it is, and make it a fun thing to do. You can win from any position on the board, as you are the creator of your life.

Q   There is an orgasmic "forest" through which it is difficult to see the trees. Just a century ago the nonorgasmic woman was considered normal. Nowadays a "one-shot orgasm" woman is seen as almost sexually retarded. Are we not forgetting the woman and the man behind the orgasm? Aren't we putting too much pressure on both of them, especially the woman?

A   One of the basic ingredients in producing a great orgasm is attention. Attention has to be on the entire person for it to be effective, and you have to recognize that each person is an individual. It doesn't work well to treat every woman or man as simply a body or machine on which you perform exactly the same steps or apply exactly the same formula. You have to look at them and feel them in their entirety. That is, besides placing great focus on their genitals, you have to feel their energy level and to notice their emotional attitudes and resistances. Each person is indeed an individual, and, physically and psychologically, everyone is unique. No two clitorises are alike, nor are any two penises. If you apply the same formula to each person, you do miss the trees for the forest.

That said, there are some specific techniques that, when properly applied, enhance the orgasm as well as the pleasure of the whole experience. Most have to do with good communication and confidence and trusting one's own integrity about what is actually happening. So, if something doesn't feel great to you—even though your partner might say how wonderful it is—you know that your encounter could be better.

People who experience great orgasms attain this state by appreciating and verbally acknowledging the pleasure they are having. This is especially important if a person wishes to go higher: the more a person can truthfully appreciate, the higher she is able to go. Appreciation also validates her partner: he feels like a whole person, and doesn't feel "forgotten."

People choose to put pressure on themselves. Sometimes this can help them feel more or do more, and sometimes it can work in reverse, creating stress. We recommend that when students first do the exercises in our books or courses, they take pressure off themselves by deliberately disallowing themselves to have an orgasm. That is, when they masturbate, we specifically tell them to do it for the pleasure of the moment; if they start to climax or ejaculate, they are actually doing their homework improperly. The goal is to peak themselves close to orgasmic freefall but to stay just on this side of the mountaintop. This enables them to keep raising their mountaintop to a higher altitude and reduces any pressure they might feel to have an explosive or massive orgasm. Once they become adept at this game, we introduce them to the concept that orgasm is our natural state—that you actually have to move your attention away from your genitals in order *not* to feel orgasmic. This relaxed way of reaching orgasm gets better and better with practice.

Orgasm is natural and is available to everyone. We have not found any students, male or female, who were unable to experience this pleasure with hand-to-genital stimulation. When it comes to genital-to-genital stimulation, however, it is a different story. The clitoris may not be stimulated with intercourse, and in those cases the woman is usually nonorgasmic.

The most pressure around sex—which most people consider inter-course—arises when people believe they have to do it as if they were a sexual world champion, that they are not supposed to talk or to ask any questions (some moaning is permitted), that it has to be done in the dark, and that both members are supposed to experience simultaneous orgasm.

Q Do we really have, in this ever-crazier world of ours, time for an hour-long orgasm? Happy sex is more than never-ending orgasm, isn't it?

A Who is responsible for your time? Who chooses how you divvy up your day? What are the important goals you wish to accomplish? We believe that we are responsible for creating our lives and deciding what to do. Some people spend two hours a day, or more, driving to work. Others spend hours in front of the TV. Many folks spend many minutes arguing and fighting with each other. Some people spend hours preparing food. We are not saying any of these habits are good or bad, but many people do feel victimized by time; they feel they lack enough time for what they really want to do. The best way to take control of your life is to first agree with it. Realize that you set yourself up to do what you do, and that nobody is holding a gun to your head and making you do it.

As far as a one-hour orgasm is concerned, there is plenty of time in a day, twenty-four hours at least, but we don't recommend that an hour-long orgasm is what people "should" do. We demonstrate a one-hour orgasm in our courses only to show that it is possible and that there are no limitations on how long we can feel pleasure or how much pleasure we can feel. Most people have orgasms, if they have them at all, for a few seconds or a few contractions; the one-hour orgasm simply demonstrates the possibility that there is something (a great deal, in fact) more to look forward to. This does not mean you have to duplicate it in order to have a sensational life or sex life. The usual orgasm that we do in the privacy of our own bedroom lasts about ten to twenty minutes. It starts with the first stroke and continues until the end of our encounter.

Once you have experienced an extended massive orgasm, you will no longer doubt your ability to have one. You will become more grounded in your daily activities, and you will no longer feel uncertainty about your body's sexual response capabilities. You do not have to have an EMO every day, although that could be fun. Because a great orgasm has to be fueled by great communication, its benefits are many: it builds intimacy, and that is what is responsible for your feelings of happiness and love—all the wonderful physical sensations and contractions are a byproduct of this intimacy.

Q At what time in life is a women the most (and the least) orgasmic? Is there a time in one's life when one should stop "doing it"?

A We have not found an age at which women were unable to have orgasms. We have taught women in their seventies and men in their eighties who were able to have and give an EMO. As long as blood is flowing to the genital region, no reason exists why a person cannot experience great pleasure unless the nervous system has been damaged. Even if there are some circulation problems, the genitals can still feel pleasure without being engorged.

Usually, the younger the woman—say, in her twenties or teens—the less interested she is in having great orgasms. She becomes more interested in orgasm with each decade after that. We have known a few women who learned to have EMOs in their early twenties. Although this is not usual, it does show that a woman who is interested can have great orgasms even at this early age. Likewise, although a woman may experience a decline in sex hormones as she passes menopause, many postmenopausal women also embrace a liberated attitude that causes them to desire sensual pleasures more than younger women do. So EMOs depend more on attitude than on any age-related response. The strength of the orgasm does not correlate with a person's age, and a woman at any age can have an EMO. It is really a decision the woman makes about how high a priority she puts on wanting one.

There is a time and a place for an orgasm. If you are recovering from abdominal surgery, you may not want to have strong contractions in your abdomen, or if you are presenting a paper in class, you may not want to be in the throes of an intense orgasm at the time. So there may be specific times or moments in your life when you do not wish to be orgasmic, but no age exists when our sexual appetites dry up, unless we let them.

Q What are your comments on a real-life orgasmatron [a hypothetical machine that, as in Woody Allen's movie *Sleeper,* can produce endless orgasms]?

A We do not know of any real-life orgasmatrons, even vibrators. We have found in our research that women who use vibrators usually have difficulty experiencing orgasm when they switch to manual stimulation. Their orgasms are better—that is, more intense and longer—after they've stopped using the vibrator for a time. The vibrator usually causes women to tense up, so that they become numb to manual touching. We recommend that women stop using their vibrators when they are exploring the far reaches of their pleasurable potentials. We think that if someone really likes her vibrator and is happy with it, it is fine for her to use it, but we will not work with her.

If a great orgasmatron were to become available, we would be open to the idea. We sometimes recommend that our women students use a water hose in their bathtubs if they wish to enjoy external stimulation without a partner. Some women also like to use the water from a bidet to stimulate their genitals. You can read more about this in the "Masturbation" chapter.

Q If I want my partner to enjoy each stroke, how slowly should I stroke? How many strokes per five seconds do you do on a woman?

A The slower the stroke, the more time one has to enjoy it. It depends a lot on what one is used to and who is doing the stroking. From our experience, it appears that women can pleasurably experience a great range of speeds on their clitorises. They may be better able to notice and describe one slow stroke as opposed to ten fast ones, but sometimes the pleasure from the many fast strokes is greater than that from the one slow one. In a typical session, we use both fast and slow strokes, and depending on the circumstances, the woman prefers one speed. The next time, however, she may prefer the other.

Men tend to use fast strokes on themselves and to want their partners to rub them the same way. We think men definitely benefit from going more slowly (or having their partners go more slowly) and feeling the entire gamut of each stroke. Once they are able to enjoy a slow stroke as much as or more than a fast one, they enjoy the fast strokes more, too. The penis has fewer nerve endings than the clitoris; consequently, men seem to miss more of the fast strokes than women do. The clitoris's greater number of nerve endings allows a woman to adapt more quickly to a fast stroke.

When touching someone, first remember that you are touching for your own pleasure. The speed and pressure of the stroke depend on how you feel, combined with what your partner indicates feels best to him or her. There is no right pressure and no right speed. Sometimes the appropriate stroke is really fast, and other times it can be very slow—from, say, five strokes per second to one stroke every ten seconds. Use your intention—which is your focused attention plus your strong intent—to take your partner higher. Do whatever feels best. After every peak, you can switch from a fast stroke to a slow one or from a light stroke to a firm one. Find out which one feels best to your partner and to your finger.

Q We and our wives are confused about the length of time that should be spent touching the clitoris. It gets very sensitive to the touch, and yet you say to keep touching it.

A First, remember to verbally appreciate your partner as much as you can. Also, don't forget to use lubricant when touching the clitoris. If you keep rubbing the same spot on the clitoris or anywhere else, it won't want to be touched anymore; that is why you must peak her or deliberately bring her down *before* that happens. Then you can start stroking again: because you stopped before she was quite ready, she will want more. This enables her to go higher. Also, remember that the goal is not how long you can rub but how much pleasure and fun you can have with each stroke. If you are concerned only with time spent on the clitoris, you are missing the fun.

Some women think they have super-sensitive clitorises that cannot be touched at all or that can be touched only for a short time. If this describes your wife, use lots of lubricant and touch lightly. Once she trusts you and has confidence that you will not hurt her, she will put her energy into feeling pleasure instead of resisting pain. At first, give her only a few strokes at a time, so she will want more and will be less afraid of feeling too sensitive. With practice, she will be able to feel more pleasure and to feel it for longer periods of time.

Q Can one or two glasses of wine help a woman mellow out and make her more susceptible to being done and having an EMO?

A Alcohol is a nervous-system depressant. Therefore, it could help someone relax. It also helps people with strong inhibitions to consider doing something they normally might resist. The trouble with alcohol is that if you drink more than a certain amount, it interferes with what you actually feel. Your sensations are depressed.

Therefore, we don't recommend alcohol before a "do"; but if it is used, take only small amounts—one glass of wine, at most, to help you relax and loosen up a little. We have found that the biggest and best orgasms happen not from alcohol or drugs but from real desire.

~ Bibliography ~

Angier, Natalie. *Woman: An Intimate Geography.* New York: Houghton Mifflin, 1999.

Asbell, Bernard, with Karen Wynn. *What They Know about You.* New York: Random House, 1991.

Baranco, Vic. *Things I've Heard Vic Say,* vol. 6. Lafayette, CA: More University Press, 1991.

Bodansky, Steve, and Vera Bodansky. *Extended Massive Orgasm: How You Can Give and Receive Intense Sexual Pleasure.* Alameda, CA: Hunter House, 2000.

De Waal, Frans. *Bonobo: The Forgotten Ape.* Berkeley, CA: University of California Press, 1997.

Dodson, Betty. *Sex for One: The Joy of Self-Loving.* New York: Three Rivers Press, 1974.

Fisher, Helen E. *The Sex Contract: The Evolution of Human Behavior.* New York: William Morrow, 1982.

Friday, Nancy. *My Secret Garden.* New York: Pocket Books, 1973.

———. *Women on Top.* New York: Pocket Books, 1993.

Gleick, James. *Faster: The Acceleration of Just About Everything.* New York: Vintage Press, 1999.

Hyde, Janet S., and John Delamater. *Understanding Human Sexuality.* New York: McGraw Hill University Press, 2000.

Kodis, Michelle, David Moran, and Deborah Houy. *Love Scents: How Your Natural Pheromones Influence Your Relationships, Your Moods, and Who You Love.* New York: Penguin Putnam Press, 1998

Lowry, Thomas P., ed. *The Classic Clitoris.* Chicago: Nelson Hall, 1978. Includes "Corpus Clitoridis," by Kermit E. Krantz, about clitoral anatomy, and "The Female Sex Organs in Humans and Some Mammals," by Ludwig George Kobelt, a description of the clitoris. Krantz's article was originally published in *Obstetrics and Gynecology* 12 (1958): 382–96; Kobelt's article was first published in 1844.

Mathews, Gary. *Introduction to Neuroscience.* London: Blackwell Science, 2000.

Ornstein, Robert, and David Sobel. *Healthy Pleasures.* Reading, MA: Addison-Wesley, 1989.

Paget, Lou. *How to Be a Great Lover: Girlfriend-to-Girlfriend Totally Explicit Techniques That Will Blow His Mind.* New York: Broadway Books, 1999.

——————. *The Big O: Orgasms: How to Have Them, Give Them, and Keep Them Going.* New York: Broadway Books, 2001.

Strangers, Jean, Anne Neck, and Kathryn van Hoffman. *Masturbation: The History of a Great Terror.* New York: St. Martin's Press, 2001.

Thomashauer, Regena. *Mamagenas School for Womanly Arts.* New York: Simon and Schuster, 2002.

Wilber, Ken. *A Brief History of Everything.* Boston: Shambhala, 1996.

Yronwode, Catherine. "The Clitoris During Intercourse." Website: www.luckymojo.com/tkclitoris.html, 2001.

∽ Index ∽

MORE BOOKS ON SEXUALITY & ORGASM
from Hunter House

EXTENDED MASSIVE ORGASM: How You Can Give and Receive Intense Sexual Pleasure ... *by* Steve Bodansky, Ph.D., & Vera Bodansky, Ph.D.

Yes, extended massive orgasms can be achieved! In this hands-on guide, Steve Bodansky and his wife Vera describe how to take the experience of sex to a new level of enjoyment.

Focusing primarily on women but addressing the needs of men as well, the authors disclose knowledge that is practically unknown except to specialized researchers and involves the stimulation of specific and uniquely sensitive areas. They recommend the best positions for orgasm and offer strategic advice for every technique from seduction to kissing. No matter how long a couple has been together, it's never too late—or too early—to make each other ecstatic in the bedroom. The Bodanskys explain how.

224 pages ... 6 illus. ... 12 b/w photos ... Paperback $14.95

FEMALE EJACULATION & THE G-SPOT

by Deborah Sundahl ... Foreword by Alice Kahn Ladas

Discover the G-spot's hidden sensations of intense pleasure.

The G-Spot is a woman's prostate gland. When stimulated, it swells with blood and emits ejaculate fluid, usually during orgasm. All women have a G-Spot, and all women can ejaculate. This has been known since classical times and in the sacred sexual texts of Tantra, Indian sexual mysticism. Author Deborah Sundahl has led seminars on female ejaculation for 15 years, and this book is based on her research. Contents include:

* reasons why some women ejaculate and others don't
* techniques, positions, and aids that help a woman ejaculate
* how men can help their female partners to ejaculate

Massage techniques developed by body work specialists and Tantric healers are included along with exercises to help release emotional pain.

288 pages ... 6 illus. ... Paperback $15.95 ... Publication September 2002

SIMULTANEOUS ORGASM and Other Joys of Sexual Intimacy

by Michael Riskin, Ph.D., & Anita Banker-Riskin, M.A.

Based on techniques developed at the Human Sexuality Institute, this guide shows couples how they can achieve the special, intimate experience of simultaneous orgasm.

The first part examines research on simultaneous orgasm, the second describes specific techniques and gives step-by-step instructions to help individuals achieve orgasm separately, then simultaneously. Each exercise includes practical advice for relaxing and feeling comfortable with your own sexuality and that of your partner. A separate section explains the purpose of the exercise and offers insights about how it can positively affect your relationship. The authors also explore gender differences and the emotional rewards of achieving simultaneous orgasm.

240 pages ... 9 b/w photos ... Paperback $14.95 ... Hardcover $24.95

To order, or for our FREE catalog of books, please see last page or call 1-800-266-5592.

SEXUAL SELF-HELP FOR EVERYONE
Three Books *by* Barbara Keesling, Ph.D.

SEXUAL PLEASURE: Reaching New Heights of Sexual Arousal and Intimacy

This book is for anyone who wants to learn how to make love without anxiety or pressure. It starts from the basic lesson of intimacy: learning to explore and enjoy touching and being touched. It also encourages you to focus on your own desire rather than trying to please your partner. This puts you in touch with your body and feelings and leads naturally to greater pleasure for both partners.

Sexual Pleasure then introduces a series of unique **sensate focus** exercises, to be done alone and with a partner, to increase sensual awareness. The exercises can be used independently of sexual orientation, by those who have physical limitations, or by those who are just learning about sexuality—anyone interested in better sex.

224 pages ... 14 b/w photos ... Paperback $13.95 ... Hardcover $21.95

MAKING LOVE BETTER THAN EVER: Reaching New Heights of Passion and Pleasure After 40

Great sex is not reserved for those under 40. With maturity comes the potential for a multi-faceted, soulful loving that draws from all we are to deepen our ties of intimacy and nurturing. That is the loving that sustains relationships into later years. In this book, Dr. Barbara Keesling shows couples how to reignite sexual feelings while reconnecting emotionally. She provides a series of relaxation, body-image, and caress exercises that demonstrate the power of touch to heighten sexual response and expand sexual potential; reduce anxiety and increase health and well-being; build self-esteem and improve body image; open the lines of communication; and promote playfulness, spontaneity, and a natural sense of joy.

208 pages ... 14 b/w photos ... Paperback $13.95 ... Hardcover $24.95

Rx SEX: Making Love Is the Best Medicine

This warm and insightful book offers rare information about the restorative powers of sex. *Rx Sex* asks what you want to heal—emotions, physical problems, or a relationship—and directs you to a setting and exercises that are right for you. Adults of any age and sexual orientation can use the exercises, which progress from simple to advanced. Some of the positive effects include:

** physical benefits: strengthening your immune system, breathing and circulation; healthier skin, hair and eyes; pain relief, especially from chronic conditions

** mental and emotional benefits: helping you overcome depression and anxiety; improving concentration and memory; restoring a positive body image

192 pages ... 14 b/w photos ... Paperback $13.95

To order or for our FREE catalog call (800) 266-5592

A PORTABLE SEXUALITY LIBRARY
Four Pocketbooks *by Richard Craze*

THE POCKET BOOK OF SENSATIONAL ORGASMS

Designed for couples in loving relationships, this is a unique and informative look at how couples can intensify, extend, and enhance orgasms together. The first two sections explain the physiology of orgasm, the last four sections provide practical and stimulating exercises for partners.

By learning about techniques such as "The Tail of the Ostrich" and the "Two Hand Twist," partners release inhibitions and can share an erotic adventure. Craze also highlights topics such as why and how we orgasm; the difference between male and female orgasms; types of orgasms: vaginal, clitoral, G-Spot, anal, multiple, mutual, and oral; and how to magnify sexual satisfaction: tips for seduction and foreplay.

96 pages ... 64 color photos ... Paperback $11.95 ... Publication OCTOBER 2002

THE POCKET BOOK OF FOREPLAY

Foreplay isn't just a prelude to the "real thing"—it's an experience to be savored for itself. This book shows you how, with full-color pictures providing a guided tour of the joys of foreplay, from "Setting the Scene" to "Reaching the Limits."

Ever wanted to try foreplay at the office or fantasized about those sexy Tantric techniques? The full range of foreplay fun is here, adding an erotic new dimension to your lovemaking experience.

When a relationship falls into a routine that becomes boring, instead of looking for another lover to spice up your sex life, try experimenting with foreplay to put sparkle and excitement back into your connection.

96 pages ... 68 color photos ... Paperback $10.95

THE POCKET BOOK OF SEX AND CHOCOLATE

What more could a body want? Explore the pleasures of the ultimate combination—sex and chocolate. Treating sex as an art form, Craze's suggestions for combining chocolate and sex run the gamut from saucy to classy. Readers learn about the best kinds of chocolate—and what to do with it. How to smear, lick, dribble, and, of course, eat it. Illustrated with sensuous photographs, this book will give new meaning to the joy of chocolate.

96 pages ... 67 color photos ... Paperback $10.95

THE POCKET BOOK OF SEXUAL FANTASIES

Our imagination knows no bounds when it comes to lust, passion, and sexual possibilities. This book explores why fantasies are important and how to get beyond inhibitions and act out your fantasies, how to set limits and say "stop" without undermining the erotic moment, and how to take turns. It guides readers through all the common genres of fantasy, including bondage, striptease, voyeurism, fetishism, toys, teasing, leather and lace, exhibitionism, and cross-dressing and touches on how fantasy can become an art form or a ritual.

96 pages ... 64 color photos ... Paperback $10.95

All books may be ordered at our website, www.hunterhouse.com

ORDER FORM

10% DISCOUNT on orders of $50 or more —
20% DISCOUNT on orders of $150 or more —
30% DISCOUNT on orders of $500 or more —
On cost of books for fully prepaid orders

NAME

ADDRESS

CITY/STATE   ZIP/POSTCODE

PHONE   COUNTRY (outside of U.S.)

TITLE	QTY	PRICE	TOTAL
The Illustrated Guide to EMO (paperback)		@ $16.95	
Extended Massive Orgasm (paperback)		@ $14.95	
Prices subject to change without notice			
Please list other titles below:			
		@ $	
		@ $	
		@ $	
		@ $	
		@ $	
Check here to receive our book catalog ❏			*FREE*

Shipping Costs
*By Priority Mail: first book
$4.50, each additional
book $1.00
By UPS and to Canada:
first book $5.50, each
additional book $1.50
For rush orders and other
countries call us at (510)
865-5282*

TOTAL	_____
Less discount @_____%	(_____)
TOTAL COST OF BOOKS	_____
Calif. residents add 7½% sales tax	_____
add Shipping & handling	_____
TOTAL ENCLOSED	
Please pay in U.S. funds only	

❏ Check   ❏ Money Order   ❏ Visa   ❏ MasterCard   ❏ Discover

Card # _____ Exp. date _____

Signature _____

Complete and mail to:
Hunter House Inc., Publishers
PO Box 2914, Alameda CA 94501-0914
Phone (510) 865-5282 Fax (510) 865-4295
You can also order by calling **(800) 266-5592**
or from **www.hunterhouse.com**

IMO 5/2002